Is There a Diet for Chronic Illness?

Pati Chandler

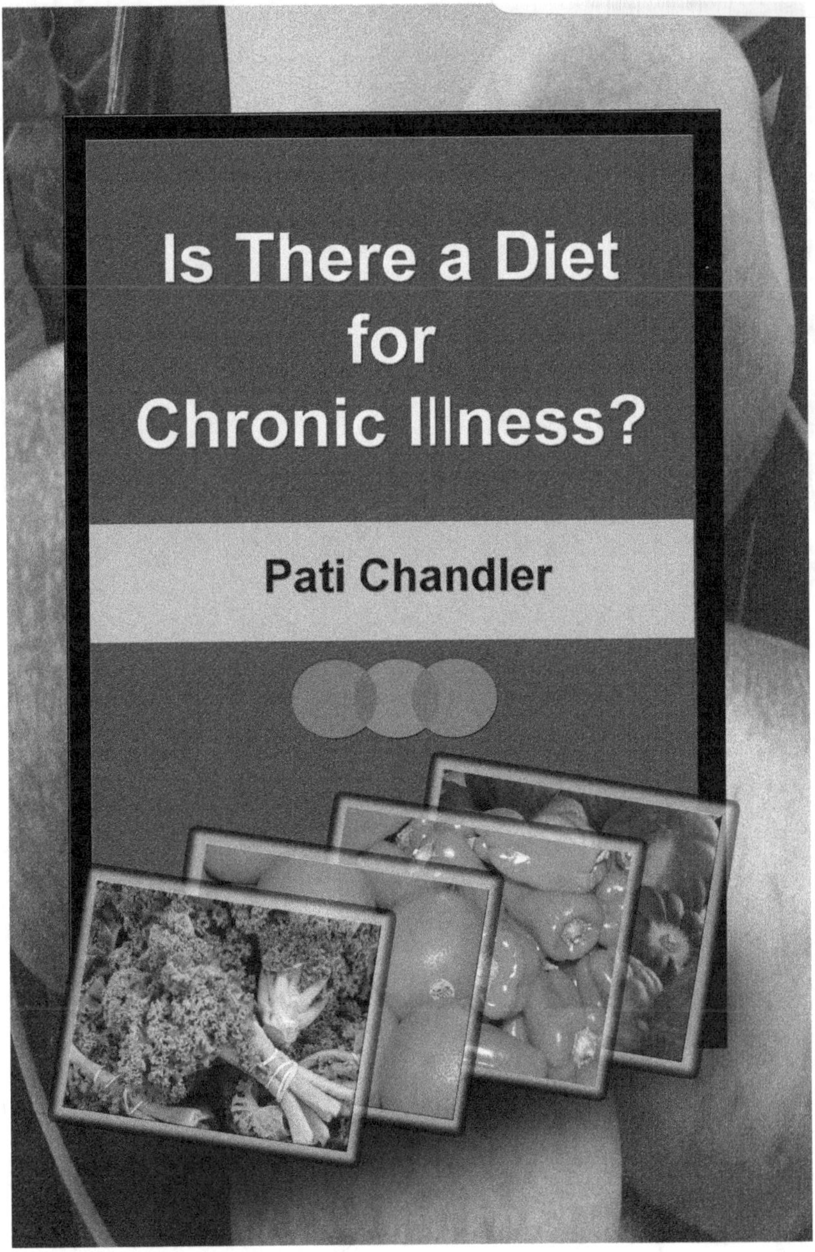

IS THERE A DIET FOR CHRONIC ILLNESS?

Pati Chandler

Copyright

Is There a Diet for Chronic Illness?
ISBN-10: 978-1496174277
ISBN-13: 1496174275
Copyright © 2014
An
I.W.A. Publishing Services project.
iwa.yolasite.com
Westborough, MA
Copyright © 2014
Library of Congress in Publication Data
Chandler, Pati
Is There a Diet for Chronic Illness?
Written by Pati Chandler
Edited by Zorina Exie J. Frey
Copyedited by Zorina Exie J. Frey
Cover Design, Photos, and graphic designs by
Zorina Exie J. Frey

Disclaimer

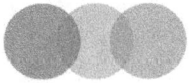

All information provided within this book is for informational and educational purposes only. It is not intended to diagnose, or treat any illness, nor is it intended as a substitution for care from a professional. Please consult your physican or a qualified health professional for advise, diagnosis, and medical treatment.

Table of Contents

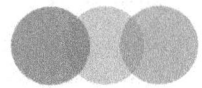

Foreword

Introduction

Preface

Part 1

Part 2

Part 3

Foreword

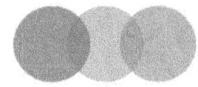

"Pati Chandler has once again distilled the essence of a complex subject and made it accessible in simple, digestible terms. The practical advice she presents will allow us all to partake of a palatable, even delicious anti-inflammatory feast."

~Kusumakar Bhatt, DO
The Mishawaka Clinic

"I would definitely listen to what this woman has to say. It would be hard to find a more knowledgeable or more caring woman in the field. I was always told in school that unless someone believes you care, they won't listen to you. Pati speaks with deep compassion and understanding. There is a wealth of knowledge in this book, and I highly recommend it to anyone interested in learning about chronic illness."

~Kevin D. Hancock, DC
University Park Chiropractic

Introduction

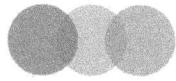

Truth be told, I believe that most people in the civilized world have forgotten the purpose of eating. We eat out of boredom, habit, nervousness, or anxiety. We eat because someone else is eating. We eat to celebrate. We eat on the run while multi-tasking. We eat for entertainment. We eat unconsciously. And we eat anything quick and handy – "on the go" foods; and the food industry has been nicely accommodating us since the first days of frozen dinners and packaged or boxed foods.

Now, all this eating is not a bad thing. After all we must eat, but it's what we choose to eat that has become the problem.

Actually, the purpose of eating is to provide nourishment, sustenance…fuel for the body. Yet, there is fuel and then there is fuel. Would you put sugar, acid, or chemicals in your gas tank? Believe it or not we put these things in our bodies on a regular basis. Fuel? For many, this kind of fuel doesn't work long before things begin to go terribly wrong—some sooner than others.

Eating healthy foods can actually be a huge part of helping to relieve pain, exhaustion, sleep, stomach issues, and countless other symptoms. Healthy foods are especially important for those with a chronic illness because they include powerful antioxidants, superb immune boosters, impressive inflammation fighters, and amazing pain terminators!

It is also true that there are a number of foods—even whole, healthy foods that can react poorly in a chronically ill body. This is just one more of those surprises that comes with your diagnosis! All of a sudden some foods may no longer be compatible with your universe. You may have been going along all your life eating certain foods, but now with your diagnosis, things have changed, rather drastically. In actuality, it isn't all of a sudden at all. It's been building up, deep inside without you're ever feeling a thing until…POW, there it is!

> **Amazingly, some or many of your muscle aches, joint pains, heart palpitations, headaches, anxiety attacks, depression, mood swings, fatigue, abdominal discomfort, bowel issues and more, may be relieved by simply avoiding or greatly minimizing certain foods!**

Reactions

The statement above may sound way too simple, I know. But you need to realize that your body is different now and it is reacting differently to the *same* stimuli. Whether that stimuli is a stressful situation, familiar foods, or a chair that is no longer comfortable; or whether it's hot or cold outdoor temperatures, loud noises, or certain odors, your body is acting, or I should say RE-acting, differently than it had in the past.

Your immune system isn't functioning on all thrusters; your mental processes closely resemble Swiss cheese; your body doesn't move the way it used to, and your nervous system seems to have a short in it. Your body is much more sensitive to a whole host of things now than it ever was before. And yes, you may have acquired some food allergies you never had before – spring, summer, or fall allergies too, for that matter.

There are foods that create fatigue; foods that create pain; foods that cause stomach issues; foods that cause nerve sensitivities; foods that can lead to depression; foods that cause inflammation and on and on. Even though these have never been an issue for you before your diagnosis, you need to understand that things have changed. Your body has changed. It doesn't react to things the same way anymore. Food sensitivities and intolerances may NOW be a very real part of your life!

Food sensitivities and food intolerances can show up in a huge variety of ways, including allergy-type symptoms such as dry, burning throat, watery eyes, runny nose, post nasal drip (throat clearing), and diarrhea. These and other symptoms may show up as the mysterious "day-later" symptoms that are indicative of a sensitivity. These may also be the same symptoms that mystify everyone because they often don't happen at the time of ingestion; they have a delayed reaction.

Reactions like fatigue, bloating, gas, mood swings, nervousness, headaches, or even muscle or joint pain often show up hours later, a day later or even two days later. So it's hard to tell exactly what caused the symptoms, and they may be viewed as a part of your chronic illness. Consequently, if these are foods that you eat every day, the symptoms may be daily and constant, further confirming the suspicion of their being a part of your illness. But what if they're a food sensitivity stemming from your chronic illness and are really something that you can relieve simply by deleting that food from your diet?

What if many of your symptoms are really caused by a food sensitivity stemming from your chronic illness, and all you have to do to relieve some symptoms is to delete certain foods from your diet?

Food Journal

This is where a food journal becomes indispensable. This is really the very best way to find out what foods are helping or hurting. If you were to write down every food, drink, or substance that passes your lips including chewing gum, then you can look back and check what you ate yesterday or even two days ago.

In your food journal there's no need to "cheat" or conveniently forget to write down that cookie you grabbed on your way out the door. This little pocket-sized spiral notebook is for your eyes only. This little book is as sacred as your medical files. No one gets to see this privileged information, not even your doctor, unless you allow it.

When you look back in this little notebook and find one or more suspicious foods that you ate yesterday or the day before, it will be worth an Elimination Test (see Info Box 1) to find out if some or many of your symptoms can be relieved, or at least greatly helped by simply omitting that specific food. It is recommended to choose only one suspicious food at a time. If you eliminate two or more, then you won't know which one is the offender. The idea is to find the offender and render it GONE along with the pain and symptoms that it was creating!

"Every time you eat or drink, you are either feeding your disease or fighting it."

~Heather Morgan, MS, NLC

Preface

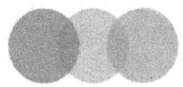

"Every patient carries his or her own doctor inside."

~Albert Schweitzer

Illness, like wellness, is a condition of the whole being – the body, the mind, and the spirit. In order to bring about wellness to an ailing body, all three must be addressed. When a head cold hits, for example, you don't consider yourself well until 1) the body feels better, 2) the mind is fully functioning and 3) laughter is once again a part of your day. This is wellness.

Chronic illness is the same, yet different. Chronic, by definition, means long term – often lifelong. Then there is chronic pain. Sometimes chronic pain is caused by a specific injury, like an accident or fall, but not always. Chronic pain also comes about as autoimmune conditions that seem to just "show up." There are more than 100 autoimmune conditions, some of which are: chronic low back pain, arthritis, migraines, fibromyalgia, Alzheimer's, multiple sclerosis, chronic headaches, Chronic Fatigue Syndrome, Lyme Disease, cancer, high cholesterol, high blood pressure, complex regional pain syndrome (CRPS), lupus, rheumatoid arthritis, Sjogren's

Syndrome, Grave's Disease, Hashimoto's Disease, diabetes, Crohn's Disease, and many more.

The body is affected of course by the pain, fatigue, and other symptoms of the specific condition. The mind is, among other things, that which processes the chemical reaction of the pain and symptoms. But, the mind is also where perception is located—the perception of the all-encompassing pain and symptoms often to the exclusion of all else. The spirit is affected, of course, by the feelings brought on by the perception. Feelings of depression, anxiety, resignation, hopelessness, lethargy, and yes, anger.

> **The idea here is that the patient must be proactive.**
> **He or she must consciously take steps to address all three –the body, the mind, and the spirit.**

Pain and depression commonly occur together. No mystery here. The chemical pathways for both are in the same side of the brain. The mind processes the chemical reaction of the pain, and depression ensues, especially if it's daily pain, taking the spirit into a downward spiral. However, it's all connected. So addressing the other side of the brain, where joy, laughter, play, contentment, serenity, peace and love reside pulls everything together to help balance things out. Putting your mind here will help neutralize the other side. It's all connected and addressing one side which will ultimately affect the other.

This is why meditation, prayer, Yoga, Tai Chi, EFT (Emotional Freedom Technique), deep breathing, music, art, nature, visualization, CBT (Cognitive Behavioral Training) and other stress-relieving techniques are so helpful for depression. They work on the other side of the brain. They lift the spirit. The spirit lifts the mind, and both of these help the body.[1]

In the medical model this is why anti-depressants are prescribed for many chronic illnesses. Pain and depression share the same biological pathways and neurotransmitters.[2] So, the thinking here is that treating depression chemically also treats the pain. Killing two birds with one stone as it were; and so it does for a time.

However, for people with a chronic illness these pathways and neurotransmitters are stuck on full throttle, 24/7. They are wide-open, with no rest in sight! No balance of rest and activity necessary for proper brain function. Sylvia Marten's article, "How Chronic Pain Leads to Depression" tells of new research results now being published by Dante Chialvo in the Journal of Neuroscience.[3]

According to Chialvo, lead author and associate research professor of physiology at Northwestern University's Feinberg School of Medicine, there may be a problem with the present method of treatment for those with chronic illnesses. Again, chronic means long-term.

"If you are a chronic pain patient, you have pain 24 hours a day, seven days a week, every minute of your life," Chialvo said. "That permanent perception of pain in your brain makes these areas in your brain continuously active. This continuous dysfunction in the equilibrium of the brain can change the wiring forever and could hurt the brain."

Chialvo's research suggests that controlling only pain may not be desirable for the long term. Rather, he feels it may be essential to study new approaches for treatment, which would include an evaluation and prevention of this dysfunction in the equilibrium in the brain.

This dysfunction in the brain means that the brain gets no rest, literally. The mind is never turned down or off. There must be a balance in all things in nature. And so it is with the brain. There must be rest time in between the frenetic bouts of perception of pain; otherwise neurons wear out, altering their connections to each other.

Where would this rest come from? It could well come from your choice to become proactive in the management of your chronic illness. As mentioned above, meditation, prayer, Yoga, and the like can give this rest.[4] These techniques, whichever one or more that you are called to try, can absolutely ease this frenetic, continuous brain activity easing depression and pain as well. It has been proven in many studies and articles including pain research centers all over the world. Any one or more of these stress-relieving techniques can benefit the physical, mental, and emotional…body, mind, and spirit.

Being proactive in your choices about the care and feeding of your body is every bit as important as your choices for mental and emotional balance. Not only can healthier food choices make the above choices and treatments easier, they can literally ease pain and many other symptoms as well! Think how pleasurable the simple act of eating a fine meal can be; physically as well as emotionally satisfying. You are addressing the other side of the brain for balance.

Proactively helping to fortify and properly nourish the body helps mental acuity and emotional well-being giving you the energy and wherewithal to utilize those same stress-relieving techniques, prayer, Yoga, Tai Chi, EFT, etc. Balance is so important to the body. It's all connected. So let's begin.

Is there a diet for chronic pain? The answer is yes. What is that diet? It's a 3-Step plan.

1. Stop feeding the fire
2. Bring back the balance
3. Start putting out the fire with healthy nutritious foods

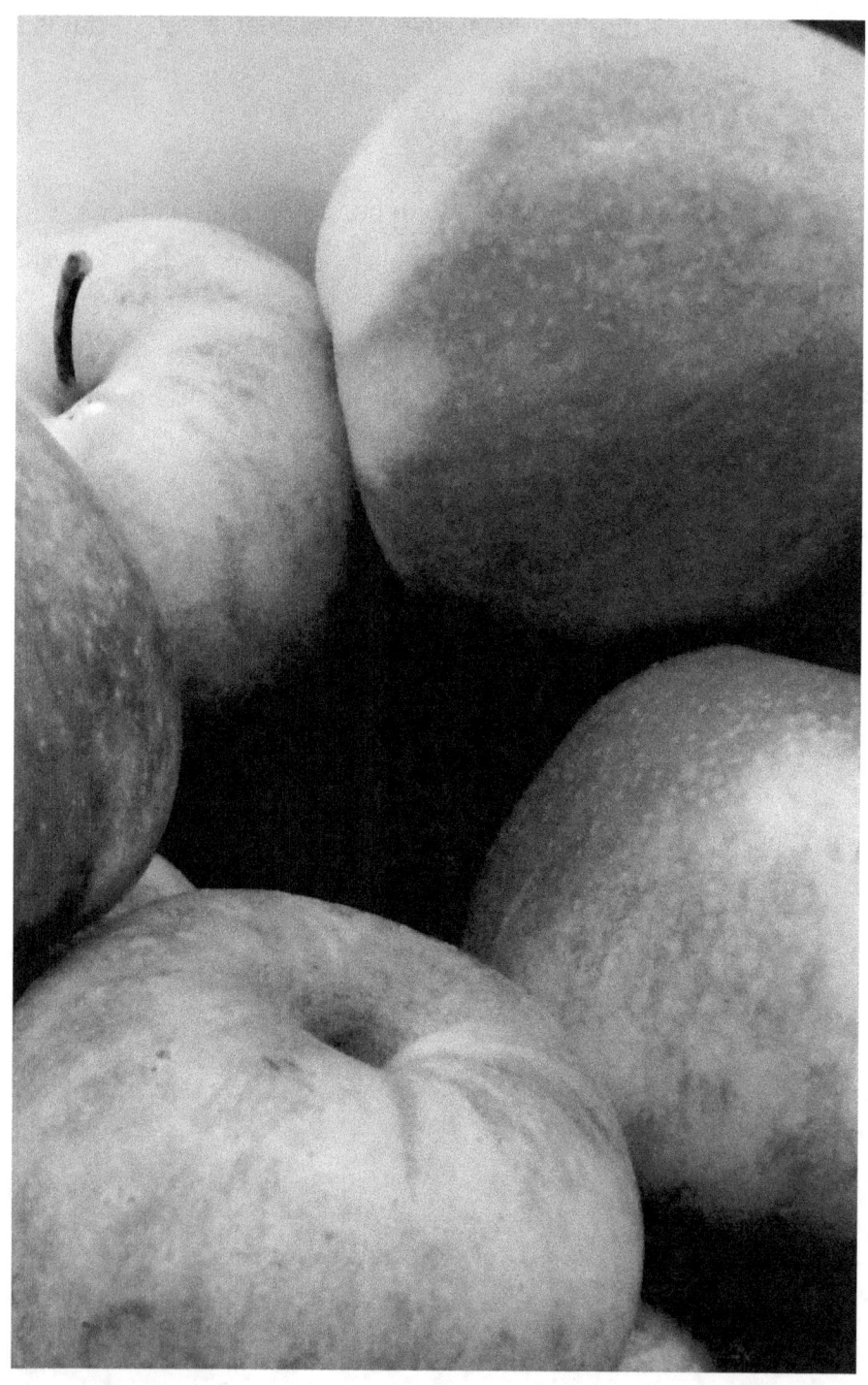

●●●

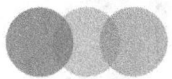

Part 1
Step One: Stop Feeding the Fire

"They always say time changes things, but you actually have to change them yourself."

~Andy Warhol

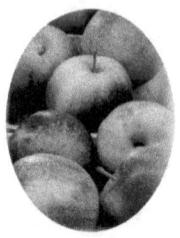

Chapter 1

A Few Words about Inflammation

According to many studies and articles, including the excellent article found at the Arizona Center for Advanced Healing, the bottom line and most likely the cause of nearly every autoimmune disease is inflammation, specifically chronic *cellular* inflammation.[1] Chronic cellular inflammation is inflammation that one doesn't *feel*; so much as reap the consequences thereof!

Inflammation is actually a very necessary and helpful natural bodily response to some form of stress—a cold, a broken finger, or a cut. This is inflammation we can feel and see, and that's a good thing. This is our immune system hard at work. We need our white blood cells to rush in with swords drawn to protect and defend the area from foreign enemies like bad bacteria and viruses.

We also need these white blood cells to protect and defend against modern day man-made toxins and "foods" that the human body was never meant to process. These man-made toxins and foods create stress on the body; and this stress calls up the inflammatory response every bit as much as a cold or a cut! Yet, we don't *see* this inflammation.

Responding as if to a 9-alarm fire, your white blood cells rush to the rescue each and every time your body is stressed to combat these foreign enemies—whether it is from a cold, a cut, lack of sleep, an inability to tolerate cold temperatures, a sudden loud noise, a gluten molecule that is impossible for your system to absorb, or a car accident. In all of these cases, there *is* stress involved and your body will activate the inflammation response for your protection, just as readily as the adrenals respond with adrenaline and cortisol.

The problem occurs when this inflammatory response is called upon day in and day out. It's accumulative, because there is no time or factor allowing healing before the next round of the inflammation signals. You may not have a cold or cut every day, but you are repeatedly exposed every day to: environmental toxins, insomnia, emotional stresses, man-made foods, foods without enough minerals and vitamins to protect a body, and drinking water with man-made chemicals like fluoride and chlorine.

Processing these things is *not* a natural function for the human body—it was simply not meant to do this. This causes stress on the body's functions and inflammation follows as a matter of course, for protection—as a part of our immune system. One can go along for years eating and experiencing these things and never know that the smoldering fires are building up and up, to a "critical mass."

Food is the key to inflammation!

Even though these experiences continually build up every single day, your body will try its best to end the inflammation and complete its job whenever it can so it can come to a balance (rest). Yet, with so many inflammation-causing factors coming at you so often, and not enough *anti*-inflammation helpers, something has got to give. Sooner or later, your body will let you know in no uncertain terms, that you just cannot continue doing this. According to the Arizona Center for Advanced Medicine, diabetes, Chronic Fatigue, arthritis, Alzheimer's, allergies, lupus, fibromyalgia, PTSD, depression, cardiovascular disease, and any other autoimmune disease that your genetics calls upon, will grab hold of you! [2]

Before 1900, our great grandparents had things under control nicely. The foods they ate were fresh whole REAL foods, full of antioxidants, minerals, vitamins, enzymes, probiotics, and so on. Consequently, their stresses were able to heal. Inflammation came, was dealt with and then went away—food heals. There were no chemical toxins put in their food or water, no bad fats, no man-made foods, no electromagnetic fields in every home, no x-rays/radiation, no gasoline fumes, no fluorescent lights, no...you get the idea! Modern society has greatly upped our exposure to inflammation-makers, and yet we have *not compensated* by upping the nutritious healing foods.

In point of fact, the modern man-made foods are adding *even more* to all this inflammation.

This inflammation is now systemic—systems wide—including the hormonal system, digestive, cardiovascular, respiratory, joint and cartilage, and it is now in a low grade smolder mode. Little clumps of white blood cells making inflammatory cytokines are clustering here and there, and they're blocking receptors in nearly every system. Vitamin D receptors, thyroid and adrenal receptors, cardiovascular receptors, digestive receptors are all looking for signals to tell them what to do, how much to send, and how much to hold back. But the communications with the brain, the gut, or the hypothalamus are either garbled or not getting there at all. This inflammation is covering the communication system!

We can take an aspirin for the aches and fever of a cold, and it takes the inflammation away. So why can't we take an aspirin (or 10) and take away this chronic inflammation?

It's because we are continually putting on more coals to try and smother the fire! What? More coals? Yes. We keep feeding the fire, literally, adding more fuel every day, every meal. It's no longer the original 9-alarm fire that your immune system is responding to, but rather a constant, incessant, persistent, smoldering bed of red hot coals. Picture the red hot, burning coals in your backyard Bar-B-Q grill.

As you are exposed to heavy metal toxicity like electromagnetic pollution, x-rays, gas fumes, chemical fumes and other toxins, in addition to emotional stress like physical pain, insomnia, and inflammation-making foods such as sugar, hydrogenated and trans fats, you are literally adding coals to your fire! Blocking receptors, garbling your internal communications, and reaching that critical mass! If you haven't already arrived!

Coming from so many sources, the one factor we have the most control over is…you guessed it, FOOD! We can *choose* foods with the necessary vitamins, minerals, enzymes, probiotics, etc. We can *choose* appropriate foods that will help fight that inflammation and all those free radicals that are being put into your body on a daily basis!

The Standard American Diet (SAD) (pitiful, actually) is not in our best interest. It is pro-inflammatory! In fact, according to Dr. Mercola, our diet is our undoing! "Despite spending twice the amount per capita on health care, the United States ranks *last* in health and mortality analysis of 17 developed nations." [3] This is completely unacceptable!

It's true there are other factors adding up to the perfect storm that instigates these chronic illnesses—stress, lack of restful restorative sleep, lowered immune function, and those things listed above. These factors may well be where the inflammation began, but we don't need to keep feeding the fire on a daily basis adding insult to injury. We can choose to be proactive and do what we can to help our bodies! Healthy foods heal!

We can be our own best health care practitioner by doing our part in keeping the fires under control by practicing stress relieving exercises, getting help for sleep issues, and so on. Our diet is one thing we can work on *right now* with almost instant results. *Food is the key*.

TIP There are tests that your doctor can order to see how much inflammation you are dealing with. One test is called a "High Sensitivity C-Reactive Protein Blood Test" (hs-CRP). It may be covered by insurance if the doc orders a cholesterol test with it. The hs-CRP level is used as a marker for inflammation in the arteries. Another test that can indicate inflammation is the fasting blood insulin level test. This test is used to screen for diabetes, but it also indicates inflammation. The higher the insulin level, the higher the inflammation.[4]

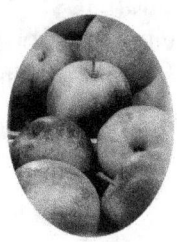

Chapter 2

Stop Feeding the Fire

The human body is a natural miracle—its workings infinitely more complex than the universe itself and in many ways still just as mysterious. We know everyone needs certain foods in order to function—foods like proteins, fats, and carbohydrates. And we know that these foods are necessary because they contain the essential vitamins, minerals, amino acids, enzymes, probiotics, and antioxidants that enable the body to function like our finely tuned, well-balanced universe. No *one* of these components is any more important than the other; they are all necessary, each in their own appropriate measure.

Yet, many of the food choices out there do not actually provide these essentials. In fact, many of the options on the grocery store shelf are downright scary! Inflammation in a box or package! Restaurants aren't any better. Our choices can make a huge difference in our body's ability to function effectively and comfortably. Choosing foods that create inflammation is *not* in our best interest!

To find out if you have a sensitivity to any food product or if they are affecting your "new" chronically ill body, you can perform your own Elimination Test. Your doctor can perform allergy and some sensitivity tests, but you can get a head start with many items, like soft drinks, artificial sweeteners, MSG, gluten, lactose etc, and specific suspected foods.[1]

Elimination Test

Stop eating or using the suspected product for one week. Notice how you feel after that time. Then begin slowly re-introducing a small serving of the item again for one day, and then another, and see how you feel. Most folks will find a noticeable difference after stopping the use of the item and decide not to do the last part of the test. OK. If your pain is a lot less, simply don't use it anymore! Be aware however, that aspartame and other tested items can be found hiding in all sorts of things. Be sure you have totally eliminated the substance from your diet even when it's in good things like yogurt or, after consulting your doctor, medications. Also, if the item has become an addiction, that is, you simply cannot stop using it for one week, then that alone should tell you the item is not in your best interest. Sugar and soft drinks are quite popular in this category. Tell your doctor if there was a noticeable difference in your pain after the above test, so s/he can have this information on file.

Info Box 1

Inflammation-Makers

Excess Sugar

Contrary to popular belief, sugar is not a food group – not even close. Don Colbert, MD, author of *The Seven Pillars of Health* (Siloam 2007), explains that sugar in its natural state, i.e. within fruits and vegetables, is quite healthy. Sugar in these foods is combined with natural fibers, vitamins, minerals, enzymes and so on to help prevent insulin spikes and excessive release of insulin in the body.

When sugar is extracted from its natural state, then refined and processed to within an inch of its life, it has absolutely zero nutritional value, and it becomes a powerful inflammation-maker! This is the sugar that is used willy-nilly in everything from cereal to ketchup, from crackers to packaged meats, from soups to processed fruit juices, and everywhere in between. *This* is when it becomes hazardous to your pain threshold, not to mention your capacity for inflammation!

Refined sugar triggers your body's reward system. The more you eat, the more you want. This is because sugar releases opioid-type chemicals in the brain that stimulates the desire for more sugar! This is a merry-go-round that is best avoided if relieving pain is a goal for you.

Sugar gives you a burst of energy for that momentary pick-me-up you may want, but the minute the sugar begins waning in your body, you *must* put more in. Sugar creates extremely *short-term* energy. This is why one soft drink is usually followed by another; one cookie is followed by another; one piece of chocolate; one jelly bean; a spoonful of ice cream…you get the idea. You only become temporarily satisfied with this dose. And if you go too long between your "something sweets," you may begin demonstrating withdrawal symptoms –becoming agitated, irritable, tired, weak, headachy, clumsy, shaky. It's amazing how a piece of chocolate, a bite of a cookie, or a sip of a soft drink *almost instantly* stops the symptoms. It's almost like magic, feeding the addiction. However, it is a *temporary* energy fix, until the next energy fix.

One of the numerous things that is happening during this temporary fix is that the sugar is interfering with the action of magnesium and calcium in your cells, limiting the production of that all-important energy molecule, adenosine triphosphate (ATP), which makes the *real*, long-lasting energy you need that comes from real food. Sugar gives that short-term boost, then it lets you down, and you need more...NOW! The sugar energy is so temporary, that you must keep inputting to continually get that boost—like a roller coaster ride. Your *real* energy, from ATP, is severely hampered by this constant sugar input.

Sugar also interferes with hormonal activity, immune function, proper protein absorption, and more. It feeds bacteria and yeast growth leading to infections; it increases fermentation in the colon and compromises your ability to fight off a cold or flu.

Nancy Appleton, PhD, author of no less than nine books on the effects of sugar on the human body, has listed 141 reasons why sugar ruins your health, complete with medical documentation.[2]

When reading food labels, check how much sugar is in a single serving of the item. Also, check the list of ingredients for sugar's many aliases. Look for ingredients ending in "ose," such as maltose, sucrose, dextrose, glucose, or fructose. Other names for sugar include high fructose corn syrup, invert sugar, beet sugar, cane sugar, corn sweetener, fruit juice concentrates, syrup or raw sugar, and of course honey or molasses. If the label lists two or three of these names, forget it. Put the item back on the shelf.

Also look to see if sugar is one of the top two or three items on the list. All ingredients are listed in order of amounts, the largest amount of something being at the top of the list, the smallest amount at the bottom of the list. If the first or second item is sugar, or if there are three different types of sugar in it, put it back on the shelf.

Soft Drinks

Soft drinks may very well rank as the number one aggravator of existing chronic pain. They also assist in the creation of a number of autoimmune conditions. Sugar is a factor of course, as is the aspartame in the diet drinks, but the phosphates in soft drinks are among the worst aggravators of pain.

Regular intake of phosphorous (phosphoric acid) can result in, not only an excess of phosphorous which depletes calcium, but also creates a potassium deficiency. When there is a deficiency of even one mineral, let alone *two*, this can render other minerals useless and inabsorbable—magnesium, for example. Therefore, what few minerals you have left become practically non-functioning.[3] This causes pain in a BIG way— both muscular pain *and* nerve pain. Your body really, *really* needs magnesium…and calcium and potassium and all the rest! Balance is the thing!

You can see where, over time, if you continue to lose these minerals daily, and don't input enough to "match" the loss, your muscles, brain, bones, etc. would slowly, but steadily become insufficient in these minerals, creating pain all the way. Information on the Natural News website quotes 18 professionals regarding soft drinks. [4]

A little trivia:

1. Containing 13 teaspoons of sugar (about 40 grams), one 12-ounce can of cola provides *nearly double* the recommended daily intake of sugar, which according to the American Heart Association should be no more than

6-9 added teaspoons per day. [5]

2. It takes up to 32 glasses of alkaline water (pH 7.5 - 8) to neutralize the phosphoric acid in just *one* can of soda pop! [6]

3. Soft drinks neutralize the enzymes in your saliva and reduce the secretion of hydrochloric acid in the stomach thereby greatly hindering digestion and mineral absorption. This also creates an atmosphere where dangerous bacteria, yeasts, and other parasites in food can thrive in the stomach! [7]

Aspartame and sugar substitutes

Aspartame is an excitotoxin. Excitotoxins are amino acids that serve as neurotransmitters in the brain. Our brains use *minute* amounts of excitotoxins for successful transmitting – one cell communicating with another. When we input *mega* doses of these excitotoxins into our body—our brain, specifically—the cells actually become so overly excited and fire their impulses so rapidly that they can actually excite themselves to exhaustion and eventually die. Dead brain cells are *not* a good thing! This hyper-activity of the cells increases your sensitivity to pain!

Aspartame, aka the pink or blue substitute sugar packets, is most often found in diet drinks and diet or "low sugar" or "sugar-free" foods. [8]

Aspartame is put into yogurt, instant breakfasts, multivitamins, instant tea, chewing gum, laxatives, wine coolers, cocoa mixes, prescriptions, OTC medications, some multi-vitamins and much more! See Dr. Mercola's website to find out where else they put it! [9]

Some of the symptoms found in people who have a sensitivity to aspartame are headaches, mood swings, depression, changes in vision, nausea, diarrhea, sleep disorders, chest pains, confusion, *increased* appetite, weight *gain*, joint pain, muscle pain, and more. Sound familiar? H.J. Roberts, MD, FACP, FCCP, Director of the Palm Beach Institute for Medical Research has coined the term, "aspartame disease" to refer to the numerous symptoms he has documented in his many articles, letters, and books on the subject of aspartame. [10]

According to some medical studies, aspartame has been linked to heart attacks, strokes, brain tumors, migraines, and seizures! [11]   It is a mystery to me why it is still on the market!

One of the most up to date websites on aspartame, MSG, and other neurotoxins is *Mission Possible World Health International.* [12]   Here you'll find news articles from around the world like, "Philippines has banned Aspartame" in Jan 2008; "Coke Zero with aspartame was banned in Venezuela due to health risks" June of 2009; and many more.

Other sweeteners. There are other sweeteners called sugar alcohols such as sorbitol, xylitol, etc. which can trigger diarrhea, along with nausea and gas (IBS). We don't even want to go there. There is saccharin which is still up in the air as to its safety. Then there is sucralose, which is made by taking away 3 of the 6 molecules in sucralose and replacing them with chlorine molecules. If you have a sensitivity to chlorine, this is necessary information. Even if you are NOT sensitive – do you really want to ingest this? [13] Also, you should know that in 2013 there were new studies on one brand name artificial sweetener that has been moved from the classification of "Safe" to "Caution" by the third party testing group, The Center for Science in the Public Interest, as told by Rachael Rettner on Foxnews.com. [14]

An Elimination Test would certainly be in order here if you are exhibiting any of the listed symptoms.

Because MSG is another excitotoxin, like aspartame, those with any chronic pain condition may indeed have a sensitivity to it. In any case it is another substance to "test" and see if this is one of the causes of your pain and other symptoms. MSG is a very common flavor enhancer, right behind salt and pepper. It is used to hide unpleasant, "off" or stale tastes.

Don't expect to find MSG on an ingredient list, however. You will need to look for any of its many aliases. [15] Here are a few of its "other" names: glutamic acid, natural meat tenderizer, "natural flavoring," yeast extract, anything "autolyzed," anything "hydrolyzed," calcium glutamate, sodium caseinate, plant protein extract, textured protein, monoammonium, and many more.

Monosodium glutamate occurs naturally in small amounts in a number of fruits, vegetables, mushrooms, meats, fish, and dairy products. But this "additive" substance, which is man-made from bacterial fermentation, is added to these same foods, multiplying the natural amount exponentially. *Then* it's added to everything else that nature never thought to put it in.

It is used in a variety of fertilizers and fungicides approved by the FDA for spraying on growing crops. MSG is found in soy sauce, Worcestershire sauce, bouillon cubes, barbecue sauces, salad dressings, seasoning mixtures, gelatin, yeast foods, etc. Under any and all aliases, it is used in abundance at all fast food restaurants and many others.

In his book, *In Bad Taste: MSG Syndrome* (Signet 1990), Dr. George Schwartz tells of some of the numerous symptoms that are identified with MSG sensitivity, such as arrhythmia, atrial fibrillation, rise in blood pressure, *migraines*, swelling, joint pain, muscle pain, chest pain, nausea, runny nose, blurred vision, numbness, diarrhea, flushing, and many more.

Dr. Russell Blaylock, famed neurosurgeon, author and

foremost authority on excitotoxins, was interviewed by Health Ranger, Mike Adams for *Natural News TV* in March of 2012. Dr. Blaylock said that the obvious symptoms seen in people with "MSG Syndrome" were "flushing of their face, heart palpitations, sometimes pain going down their arms and episodes of GI discomfort and diarrhea.... But over time, we saw destruction of major portions of the brain—things that could cause Alzheimer's disease, Parkinson's" and other brain ailments. [16]

Weight gain is another one of the very common side-effects of MSG. According to the American Journal of Clinical Nutrition, studies of a group of 10,000 healthy Chinese adults, resulted in the following conclusion: "MSG consumption was positively, longitudinally associated with overweight development among apparently healthy Chinese adults." [17]

For more information on these and other excitotoxins visit the *Mission Possible World Health International's* website. [18]

Chemical Additives

A food additive is a non-nutritive substance added deliberately to any food product to improve its color, texture, flavor, or shelf life. There are many food additives, preservatives, flavorings, and dyes which can *and do* cause a variety of symptoms and *pain* in those who are sensitive.

Some of these additives are: nitrites (in hot dogs, bologna, sausage, packaged meats), sulfites (to keep cut fruits & veggies from discoloring), sorbates, BHA & BHT (food preservatives used to keep their fats from turning rancid), and food dyes with names like "Red 40" and "Yellow 5 Lake" and "Blue 1," which of course are found in practically *everything*! *Med India* is an excellent place to begin learning of these chemical food additives. [19]

At the *Center for Science in the Public Interest*, at cspinet. com, there is a complete list of all food additives, with listings under the headings: "Safe," "Cut Back," "Caution," "People Should Avoid," and "X- Avoid." [20] Not surprisingly the items listed in the previous paragraph are found in the last two categories.

There are many studies and articles telling of children with ADHD reacting badly to food dyes. These dyes contribute substantially to hyperactivity, restlessness, and attention problems in these children. Furthermore, studies suggest that removing these dyes from the children's diet is one quarter to one half as effective in reducing these symptoms as giving these kids stimulants! In other words certain kids with ADHD might not need drugs at all if the artificial dyes were removed from their diets. Food dyes affect their neurology; and they can affect *ours* as well! One of many articles on the dangers of food dyes can be found on Dr. Oz's website, under the title "Food Dyes: Are They Safe?" [21]

It's clear that a certain percentage of the population, not only children, does indeed have a sensitivity to some or many of these additives even though they are declared safe for the majority. The idea is to find out through the old reliable Elimination Test to see if one or more of these substances may be causing some of your symptoms.

Gluten

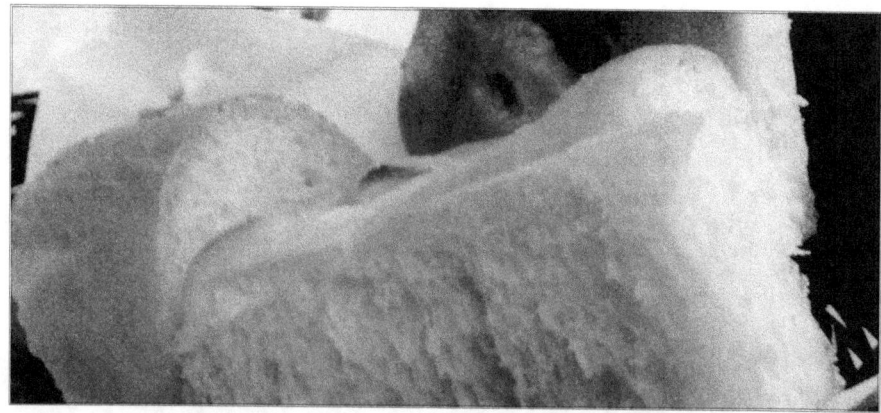

Gluten is found in the seed or kernel of wheat, barley, and rye. Oat products are often cross-contaminated with the gluten protein in processing plants, but oats do not actually have this particular protein within. The tricky part of this little bit of grain is that it is found in so *many* processed and packaged foods—a huge percentage of foods, in fact.

Gluten is obviously found in wheat or rye bread, pasta and cereals, but it is also found in beer! Gluten is injected into sausage, cold cuts, hot dogs, salami, and self-basting turkeys. It's in pita bread, flour tortillas and wraps, breadcrumbs, bagels, pizza crust, soups, puddings, yogurt, and wine coolers. It can also be found in Bourbon Whiskey. Barley enzymes are used to process chocolate chips, coffee, and dessert syrups. Gluten is used as a stabilizer and thickener in products like ice cream, custard, and gravy. As if that's not enough, it's also used as a binding agent in medications, prescriptions, and supplements. The stuff is downright hard to get away from! To find a list of "hidden sources of gluten," check out WebMD.com, or the Mayo Clinic's website. [22, 23]

Why is this a concern?

Sayer Ji, author of *The Dark Side of Wheat: New Perspectives on Celiac Disease and Wheat Intolerance* (2008), lecturer and founder of GreenMedInfo.com has written an article titled, "Wheat: 200 Clinically Confirmed Reasons Not to Eat It," where he lists these 200 medical conditions associated with gluten toxicity, complete with medical studies and related articles! Some of these are: diabetes, multiple sclerosis, chronic fatigue, infertility, schizophrenia, diarrhea, Crohn's Disease, restless leg syndrome, ADD, carpal tunnel, nervous system diseases, anemia, allergies, Sjogren's Disease, Guillain-Barre Syndrome, serotonin diseases, digestive disorders, and many more. [24]

Rodney Ford, MD, MB, BS, FRACP (Fellow of the Royal Australasian College of Physicians – in Pediatrics) of Christchurch, New Zealand, has written an article titled,

"Gluten: Bad for Us All!" where he literally presents the evidence of the universal harm of gluten.[25] Dr. Ford says, "Gluten is an important trigger of Autoimmune Disease," and then he lists diseases such as Ulcerative Colitis, Hashimoto's Thyroiditis, rheumatoid arthritis, and diabetes. Evidence is rapidly accumulating that shows gluten can severely affect our brains, nerves, and minds. The links between gluten and the brain has been extensively reviewed in Dr. Ford's book, *Full of it! The shocking truth about gluten – the brain grain connection (RRS Global Limited, 2005)*.

William Davis, MD, a preventative cardiologist and author of the New York Times bestseller, *Wheat Belly: Lose the Wheat, Lose the Weight, and Find Your Path Back to Health* (Rodale Press, 2011), calls wheat, "the perfect, chronic poison." His role as preventative cardiologist allows him to practice a unique approach to diet that allows him to advocate reversal, not just prevention of heart disease. When people stop eating gluten, he "sees diabetics become no longer diabetic; people with arthritis having dramatic relief; and people losing leg swelling, acid reflux, irritable bowel syndrome, depression and on and on every day." [26]

Grains, especially wheat, had once been known as the "staff of life." And this was quite true in the days when we carried a staff! Then along came progress and processing. The wheat we are eating now is nowhere close to the wheat that was considered the "staff of life." This wheat was engineered in the 1960s and 70s in order to increase yield, and has many different features than the original wheat that was indeed our main sustenance. [27]

Sayer Ji, tells that the current generation of wheat is "a hexaploid species, the byproduct of three ancestor plants becoming one, with 6 sets of chromosomes… and is capable of producing no less than 23,788 different proteins!" [28]

Proteins in general are the most difficult to digest of all foods and food particles. But of all the proteins, those found

Pati Chandler

in our modern wheat are ones that are the most offensive, specifically gluten. Gluten is actually the protein left behind after the starch has been washed away. Gluten itself is made up of two main groups of proteins: gliadins and glutenins (or glutelins).

The gliadin protein is an opiate-like peptide which binds to the opiate receptors in the brain and stimulates the appetite to the tune of eating 400 more calories per day...every single day. [29] The glutelins are made from the same sturdy disulfide bonds found in human hair and vulcanized rubber. They are in fact a polymer—an elastic protein, complete with viscoelastic properties similar to those found in HMM polymers.[30] This makes the protein as tough as bowling ball polymers.[31] These glutelins are responsible for the elasticity, toughness, and adhesive qualities of the gluten protein. Is it any wonder your body has a hard time digesting it completely?

There are many other proteins in gluten, like the glycoproteins known as lectins, which are pretty offensive too. They function much like "invisible thorns," and can cause a lot of damage to the intestines over time. They're particularly resistant to pH variations and temperatures, so they don't get digested easily either. [32]

What this means is that there's much more to gluten than meets the eye.

Gluten sensitivity is not exactly a "symptom" in chronic illnesses, but it is so often found in all of us, it may as well be listed as such! As shown above however, many medical professionals believe it's the other way around, where gluten sensitivity or toxicity *causes* the autoimmune conditions rather than appear as a symptom of it.

In fact, Dr. Rodney Ford tells us that "gluten is bad for us all!" Growing numbers in the medical profession have come to the conclusion that gluten is a *universal* toxin. Dr. Ford believes that it should be eliminated from the entire food chain! Keep in mind that he is a pediatric gastroenterologist and sees the damage gluten can do very early on! In children! He proposes this query: should we modify our bodies – millions, even billions of us – with drugs and/or vaccines to force our immune systems to react differently to gluten so we don't get sick (acquire autoimmune conditions)? OR should we modify our food back to the way it was, *before* we engineered it this way in the first place? [33] For now, it seems it would behoove us to modify our behavior, and avoid gluten.

***

Those with noticeable reactions to gluten are divided into two groups: 1) those with Celiac Disease, which is a life-long autoimmune disease that is genetically inherited, and 2) those with gluten intolerance, often called non-celiac gluten sensitivity or simply gluten sensitivity. Gluten sensitivity can develop at any point in life.

Celiac Disease, also called celiac sprue, is quite serious in its effect. It causes serious damage to the soft lining tissue and villi (small finger-like projections) in the small intestine which absorb the nutrients for your body. After these gluten particles do their damage to these little absorbers, the small intestine literally cannot absorb nutrients properly. Health problems from lack of nutrients, and eventually even malnutrition, slowly take over. [34]

Celiac is often under-diagnosed, especially in its early stages, as the symptoms are very sneaky. Only a small percentage of people have the usual, *expected*, gastrointestinal symptoms of bloating, cramps, diarrhea, gas, constipation, heartburn, etc. Another percentage has the "odd" symptoms that are completely unrelated to the above, and still others have no symptoms at all…until later in life when they show up as something very different.

Some of the "odd" symptoms are headaches, confusion, depression, clumsiness, arthritic symptoms, ear infections, chronic fatigue, the "blahs" and more—all symptoms that can be attributed to other conditions, or even treated as their own condition. That's what makes Celiac Disease so very deceptive; it can and often does manifest as many different individual symptoms. [35]

Gluten sensitivity, also called non-celiac gluten sensitivity, is an immune response to gluten that can occur in anyone at any time, especially if there is an overload of gluten in the body. This overload can cause major problems. [36]

A mild sensitivity to gluten can lead to temporary symptoms quite similar to Celiac Disease, such as bloating, gas, diarrhea, constipation, heartburn, headaches, arthritic symptoms, depression, "fuzzy thinking," chronic fatigue and so on. The symptoms of an overload most often show up in a day or two—the mysterious "day-later" symptoms. So if you're experiencing any, or many, of these symptoms, think back (or better yet, check your food journal) to yesterday or the day before when you had biscuits and gravy for breakfast, a pastry snack, a hotdog or pizza for lunch, cookies or crackers for a snack, soup, salad with croutons, dinner rolls, spaghetti and chocolate chip cake desert for dinner. That's a *whole* lot of gluten! And painful food!

The most insidious part of it all is that we are constantly inputting gluten ... "our daily bread" as it were. How can one rid ourselves of symptoms if we are constantly adding it to our body—a slice of toast, a pancake, a cookie, a sandwich, pasta, soup, sauces, cake, yogurt, etc?

Gluten is difficult to digest in the first place, for everyone. But when there is an overabundance of it, many of these larger undigested fragments of gluten will actually work their way through the wall of the small intestine and break out into the bloodstream, creating a nasty condition called "Leaky Gut Syndrome."

Gluten is such a large particle, that when it isn't broken

down and digested, it can actually work its way between cell walls, leaving a large opening between the cells. The more gluten you eat, the greater the risk of these larger undigested fragments breaking out of the small intestine, leaving little perforations, irritation and inflammation behind, and allowing toxic undigested material to steadily seep out into the bloodstream causing massive inflammation and other nasty symptoms throughout the rest of your body.

Eating a steady diet of massive amounts of gluten products, can *and does* lead to gluten overload in no uncertain terms. It may be time for an Elimination Test. Gluten takes a long time to get completely out of your system, so eliminating it for months may be necessary! [37]

Lactose

Lactose intolerance, like gluten sensitivity, is not exactly a "symptom" in chronic illnesses, but it is so often found in all of us that it may as well be listed as such! This sensitivity, or intolerance, is actually quite common in everyone, ill or not. More than 75% of the world's population is lactose intolerant to some extent. Being lactose intolerant means your body isn't able to fully digest the milk-sugar lactose, due to an insufficient amount of the enzyme lactase, thus it is also called "Lactase Deficiency." [38]

Infants produce lactase in abundance in order to digest mother's milk. By the time a small human turns two years old, their bodies naturally begin to slow down this process, and eventually this production of lactase stops all together.

Note: Some people, particularly those of Eastern European decent, do make lactase for a while longer because of the way they raised their cows and yaks; their bodies became acclimated to drinking that type of milk and therefore produced lactase for a longer period of time. Thus, they are able to digest lactose until early adulthood. [38a]

Adults are more likely to be lactose intolerant than children. Also, certain ethnic groups such as those of African, Asian, Hispanic, Middle Eastern, and Native American decent are more likely to be lactose intolerant. Yet, only about 20% of Caucasians are lactose intolerant, no doubt due to their Eastern European ancestors.

Lactase is not absolutely essential to digest *all* dairy items. Most people can eat some cheeses and other products in moderate amounts with no problem, even small amounts of milk, especially when eaten along with others foods. It's the large amounts of lactose that create an absolute need for the enzyme lactase. The problematic items are low-fat and skim milk, both of which have *extra* lactose added to give them flavor and body, lest they be too "watery" in texture. The small amounts of milk products found in bread, pancakes, pastries, cereals, soups, even prescription medicines like birth control pills and over the counter medicines used to treat gas and stomach acid, are not usually a problem unless the lactose intolerance is severe (or if the lactose intolerance is combined with gluten sensitivity).

In most people, symptoms are usually of a mild, if uncomfortable variety consisting of bloating, gas, nausea, abdominal cramps and diarrhea. Sound familiar? Indeed, it does mimic a number of other gastrointestinal issues, from gluten intolerance to Irritable Bowel Syndrome, to stomach flu and so on. But these symptoms are a bit easier to detect, because they show up within 30 minutes to two hours after ingesting the milk product, unlike the "day-later" symptoms of Celiac Disease and other sensitivities.

Many also have a sensitivity to the protein *casein*, found in milk and milk products. Casein protein is often used in processed foods as a binder and is usually listed in the ingredients. [39] The symptoms of this sensitivity are even more uncomfortable: itchy skin, eczema, wheezing, congestion, runny nose, or watery eyes. Adding these symptoms to the lactose issues of stomach pain, gas, nausea, or bloating can really make a body massively uncomfortable!

If you find you do have a sensitivity to this protein, be certain to check the ingredients list of crackers, cereals, etc. for "casein protein" in order to be forewarned. It is a common binder in many foods.

Test for Intolerance. An easy test to see if you are lactose intolerant is to drink two full 8 oz. glasses of milk on an empty stomach, then wait for three to four hours to see if any symptoms appear. If not, then no intolerance is evident. If so, then you may have a sensitivity to lactose or casein protein. On a different day, you can try this same test with cheese or yogurt or other milk products. If you have no symptoms, then your intolerance is considered somewhat mild and mostly restricted to milk alone.

Note: Yogurt, with live active cultures, is not usually an issue unless there is a severe intolerance because of very low amounts of lactose. Also, the live active cultures will digest the lactose for you because the enzyme lactase is actually made by the culturing process and is included in the yogurt! [40]

So what are the alternatives to cow's milk? Delicious almond milk, coconut milk, or rice milk—there is no lactose and no casein protein in any of these. Many can do quite well with goat's milk also. I don't recommend soy milk due to possible interaction with thyroid issues.

Worried about lack of calcium if you don't drink cow's milk? Not necessary. Calcium is found in salmon & sardines, sea vegetables & nori, kale & leafy greens, black strap molasses & parsley, navy beans & pinto beans, oats & tapioca, almonds & walnuts, and the list goes on and on! [41]

Hydrogenated Fats and Trans Fats

All fats are not created equal; there are good fats and bad fats. And then there are good fats that have been made *into* bad fats by processing and turning them into hydrogenated or trans fats (partially-hydrogenated fats). These good fats turned bad are listed in the ingredients of the product as veggie and seed oils like corn oil, sunflower oil, safflower oil, canola oil, soybean oil, etc. They can also be listed as monoglycerides and/or diglycerides, often listed as "mono- and diglycerides" such as found on some brand name peanut butter labels (which has hydrogenated *and* partially hydrogenated oils –aka trans fats). [42]

You have probably already heard that hydrogenated fats and trans fats are not good for your body. You should also know that they are especially hard on a body in pain. This is primarily due to the fact that they add greatly to inflammation. They also *block* any beneficial anti-inflammatory prostaglandins, promoting even more inflammation. They also add bucketsful of free radicals with every bite, aiming your body head-on into Oxidative Stress! This adds even more insult to injury by compounding the free radicals in your body nearly exponentially! [43]

The hydrogenation process injects the good natural corn and seed oils with oxygen, and a little bit of nickel, platinum, or aluminum for a catalyst, and then pressurizes and cooks the blazes out of it at 500-1000 degrees for several hours. (This also oxidizes the oil of course, turning it into free radicals.) Why hydrogenate? It is necessary in order to give the product a longer shelf-life. Indeed it does. In fact, chemically this fat is closer to plastic than any kind of food fit to be consumed by humans. [44]

French fries, cookies, crackers, donuts, margarine, cheese spreads, pastries, breads, cereals, many peanut butters, candy, fried foods, fast foods, snack foods, granola bars, health food bars...hydrogenates and partial hydrogenates are everywhere. Think: **processed + packaged + prepared foods** = dangerous to your health. [45]

The primary health risks of hydrogenated and trans

fats, after inflammation and free radicals, are the clogging of arteries. They literally act like a sticky gummy substance competing with healthy blood for room in the arteries – arteries leading to the heart, to the brain, to the kidney, to the liver, etc. This is a no-win situation for healthy blood flow, especially the flow to the brain.

All this leads to Alzheimer's, Parkinson's, cardiovascular disease, immune system dysfunction, stroke, cancer, diabetes and much more—not to mention the extra inflammation it causes when the stress of slowing blood can't get where it needs to go! [46]

All in all, this has to be one of the biggest inflammation-makers, right up there with all the others. In fact, there is no first, second, or third here. All items listed here are placed right up there in First Place! And all of these foods are matter-of-factly and routinely included in our **S**tandard **A**merican **D**iet. And have you noticed how many more of us are suffering from autoimmune conditions than ever before?

> *"So many people*
>
> *with so many autoimmune conditions."*
>
> ~Pati Chandler

Sensitivities

As it happens, many of the foods that cause inflammation may very well be foods that you are now sensitive to. Some people may be more sensitive than others and feel the effects almost immediately. For others it's more of a "build-up" thing. Yet, it always comes around to get you sooner or later, in one *way* or another. You simply cannot continue eating these inflammatory foods and *not* become affected.

Having a chronic illness, by definition, means that you *are* experiencing this deep chronic cellular inflammation, even though you can't feel it. It also means that your body is now much more sensitive to many things, including those things that *cause* this inflammation, as well as certain foods that affect systems within – the nervous system or thyroid function for example.

To find out if you have a sensitivity to any food product or if they are affecting your "new" chronically ill body, you can perform your own Elimination Test. Specific suspected foods such as nightshades and goitrogens can affect arthritis-type pain and thyroid function. Popular allergy foods can be tested too. You may not have a full-blown allergy to these items, but may have a sensitivity; thus, finding it beneficial to avoid these foods anyway.

Food sensitivities and food intolerances can show up in a variety of ways, including allergy-type symptoms such as dry burning throat, watery eyes, runny nose, post nasal drip (throat clearing), and diarrhea. These and other symptoms may show up as the mysterious "day-later symptom" that are indicative of a sensitivity. These are the symptoms that mystify everyone because they often don't happen at the time of ingestion; they have a delayed reaction.

Reactions like fatigue, bloating, gas, mood swings, nervousness, headaches, or even muscle or joint pain often show up hours later or a day or even *two days* later. So it's hard to tell exactly what caused the symptoms, and they may be viewed as "a part of the chronic illness." If these are foods that you eat every day, the symptoms may occur daily and be constant, further confirming the suspicion of their being a part of your illness. But what if they're a food sensitivity *stemming* from your illness and the solution is something that you can relieve by deleting that food from your diet?

Be vigilant with your food journal and check it frequently when experiencing symptoms!

Nightshades

Nightshade plants contain alkaloids like solanine, glycoalkaloid, etc., which can impact the nerve-muscle function, joint function, and digestive function. These alkaloids and others that are found in the nightshade family of foods have been shown to cause inflammation, muscle spasms, stiffness, and painful and inflamed joints within some people.

The family of nightshades consists of: white potatoes (*not* sweet potatoes) · tomatoes · bell peppers, red and green · sweet and hot peppers (chili peppers) · eggplant · tomatillos (commonly called green tomatoes in Mexico) · pimentos · paprika ·tobacco and others. [47]

Many people who are sensitive to nightshades can ingest small amounts with no negative effects at all, but larger quantities, or repeated quantities where it "builds up," can be highly irritating. Solanine (Solanaceae), which is found in higher concentrations in the green parts of the ripe or unripe nightshade or the green spots in potatoes, is especially toxic if consumed in large amounts. It can cause irritation and inflammation at the nerve endings and joints for sensitive people. Even cooking doesn't destroy this toxic alkaloid.

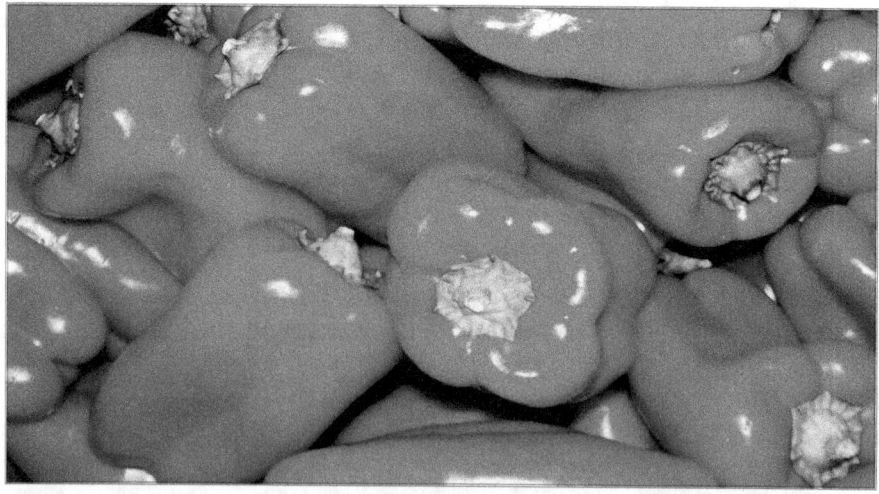

Norman Childers, PhD discovered that his own arthritis was greatly aggravated by the buildup of these alkaloids. In a 1993 study by Dr. Childers published in the *Journal of Neurological and Orthopedic Medical Surgery*, he reported that "rigid omission of Solanaceae, with other minor diet adjustments, has resulted in positive to marked improvement in arthritis and general health." [48]

According to Norman D. Ford, author of *18 Ways to Stop Arthritis Now* (Keats Pub, 1997), "...some 30% of people with genuine rheumatoid arthritis experience some degree of improvement after they eliminate nightshade foods from their diet."

Many who have fibromyalgia, arthritis, or other chronic illnesses, may suffer a sensitivity to these particular alkaloids in a similar fashion. Perform your own Elimination Test, being careful to check labels for hidden nightshades in packaged foods like soups and frozen, prepared, or boxed foods. You must eliminate ALL nightshades for a proper test. Then, after week or so, re-introduce potatoes, for example. Eat a reasonable-sized serving of potatoes at *one* meal, each day, for several days. If you have no problems, that's great. Then, omit the potatoes again and wait a couple of days. Reintroduce tomatoes in the same way. Do the same with green peppers.

You may do just fine with each food by itself. It may be that a combination or an excess of these foods that may cause the sensitivity. Combining potatoes, tomatoes, and green peppers at one meal, or all in one day, may be your undoing. Many will get along just fine by limiting the amount of nightshades they eat, and stick to only one nightshade per day or per meal. Never combining two or more at any one meal may be just the ticket.

With all the good vitamins, minerals, enzymes, and such in these foods, it would be a downright shame to have to delete them altogether. But, if you experience joint pain, muscle pain, or nerve pain of any kind, delete these foods and call it a sensitivity! Deleting or greatly limiting them may be your key.

If it's a mild sensitivity and you find no problem with eating one of these foods per day or per meal, you *can* have your potatoes and eat them too! Do it wisely if you are sensitive to these alkaloids. Don't forget, symptoms may appear later that day or even two days later! Check your food journal.

Goitrogens

This is a funny sounding word, to be sure, but if you have a thyroid issue, particularly hypothyroidism or Hashimoto's Disease, you'll need to know about it. Thyroid issues in one form or another, including goiter, are commonly found in those with autoimmune conditions.

Goitrogens are substances in certain foods that can affect the function of the thyroid gland. Don't panic. Like nightshades, limiting your amount of these foods may be all that's needed. Also, the offending chemicals in the goitrogens can be minimized with steaming, cooking or fermenting. [49]

The main goitrogens are soy and soy products like edamame and tofu, and cruciferous vegetables like broccoli, Brussels sprouts, cabbage, cauliflower, collards, kale, mustard greens and turnips.

Other goitrogens are millet, radishes, spinach, and… peanuts, peaches and strawberries! Oh no! But again, remember that limiting your quantities may be all that's needed! Whew! I'd really hate to miss out on all the antioxidants, vitamins, and minerals in these last three! Also, according to Dr. Marcelle Pick, consider gluten as a potential aggravator here too. [50]

Certain soy isoflavones, especially the one called genistein, compete with the thyroid hormone for iodine. Genistein often wins the competition, taking the iodine; or it may block the action of thyroid peroxidase. Either of these actions will leave your thyroid wanting.

If you're a fan of soy, don't give up. Steaming, cooking, or fermenting soy can pretty much mute these isoflavones, or at least render them minimally disruptive. So, foods like miso, natto, or tempeh, etc. may be fine in limited doses. Yet, it is wise to remember that soy is found in a lot of processed foods. Check the ingredients list for items like "textured vegetable protein," "isolated soy concentrate," "soy lecithin," "soy protein isolate," and others. If you are eating lots of these foods, and then add your own soy products, you are probably getting too much; thus, affecting how your thyroid functions.

Note: Be certain to have your doctor check, not only your thyroid- TSH, T3 and T4 - but your iodine level as well.

Isothiocyanates. Now there's a word! These compounds are found in cruciferous veggies and can disrupt thyroid signals as well as interfere with thyroid peroxidase in a fashion similar to genistein. But again, steaming or cooking can help minimize the effect by muting these isothiocyanates. So, cooked or steamed broccoli or cauliflower would be better than raw, for example. As for steamed peaches or strawberries? I don't think so. I'll just control myself. Peanuts? I'll do peanut butter – without hydrogenates of course, like *Smart Balance*® or *MaraNatha*® Organic, or any natural all-peanut peanut butter. But then I am also fond of almond butters.

Goitrogens are foods to be aware of, and performing an Elimination Test may be a good idea if you have a question about their effect on you and your chronic illness. [51]

Latex Foods

Latex foods? Yes, indeed. "It is estimated that 50-70 % of latex-allergic people have IgE antibodies cross-reactive to the antigens coming from some vegetable foods." [52] What does this mean? It means that anyone who may be allergic to the obvious latex found in rubber gloves, rubber bands, plastic

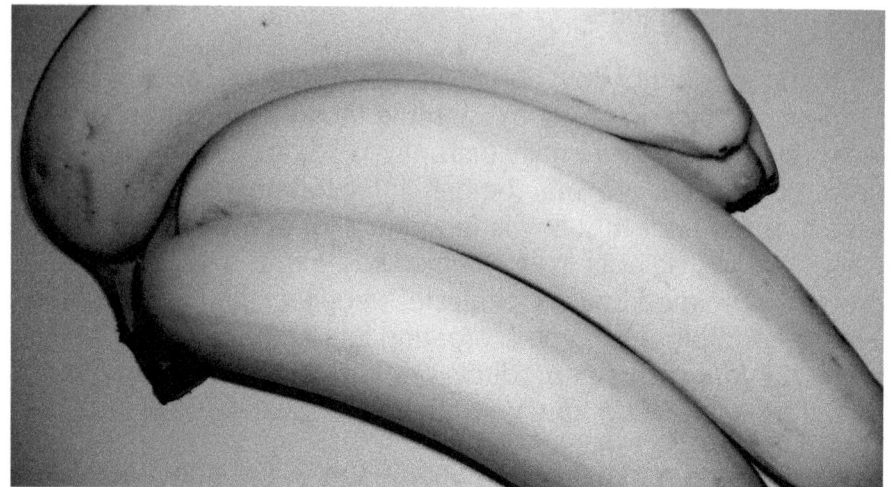

tubing, clothing, toys, floor coverings, erasers, etc. will most likely be allergic to certain foods that have a similar protein.

Even though less than an estimated one percent of the population is allergic to latex, more and more people are becoming sensitive to it due to repeated exposure, especially in health care professions, for example. [53]

Latex comes from the milky sap of the rubber tree, *Hevea brasiliensis*. One school of thought is that immediate reactions to contact with this rubber are most likely from the protein found in this plant, while delayed sensitivity reactions to these objects are usually considered to be from additives or stabilizers used to make the product. [54] However, many believe that the protein itself is the only instigator, and it's the repeated use of it that leads to a sensitivity, rather than an actual allergy. [55]

Some of these sensitivities may appear as uticaria (fancy name for a skin rash), itching, runny nose, chronic phlegm issues, difficulty breathing, and bronchial asthma. Some may even have the most severe, but rare, actual allergy and suffer anaphylactic shock from exposure to latex. [56]

So what are some of these foods which have a similar protein that you may be sensitive to? The four major offenders are bananas, avocados, chestnuts and kiwi. Some of the moderately offending foods are papaya, potatoes, tomatoes, celery, carrots, and apples. There is a low risk for other foods as well. Check The American Latex Allergy Association's website for a full list. [57]

Your sensitivity may be similar to others listed above, in that limiting your intake may be all that's necessary. Nevertheless, I highly recommend deleting these foods all together for at least a week, and then perform the Elimination Test to be sure. You might also suggest this possibility to your doctor and request an allergy test to be on the safe side.

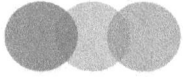

Part 2
Step Two: Bring Back the Balance

"The key to keeping your balance is knowing when you've lost it."

~Anonymous

Here we have the chicken and the egg conundrum. When you become ill, your systems go out of balance, OR when your systems go out of balance, you become ill. Both are correct. The fact is, when you are ill, your systems and components *are* out of balance. How they get that way is the million-dollar question. Often, it's due to food—inappropriate food at that. The objective is always to bring these systems and components back into balance, and back to the healthiest you that you can be. That's hard to do when the food choices available are clearly not in our best interests!

A chronically ill body uses up much of its resources to fight the illness on a daily basis. When a body is weak from this daily fight it has a difficult time "catching up" to your normal.

Your body manufactures a number of specific chemicals that naturally decrease as you age. That is, your body begins making less and less of them as a natural part of aging. This is not normally a problem for a *healthy* body because it happens a little at a time, and a healthy body can easily adapt and work fairly well with these lesser amounts.

However, if your body is in a constant and chronic state of pain and illness, many of these chemicals are still needed in sufficiently helpful quantities, and this lesser amount that your body is now making is now used up much faster in an attempt by the body to affect its own healing. There is not much chance that the body will be strong enough, have enough of the proper nutrients, or be physically able to replenish its depleting stores unless you choose the foods that will actually feed your body the required nutrients to rebuild and fortify what your body needs.

If you are feeding your body foods that deplete these helpful nutrients or compromise their actions, then the cost may well be inflammation, malfunctioning systems, and the aggravation of an autoimmune condition. Yes indeed, certain foods can and do create inflammation, pain, sleeplessness, stomach issues, and much more. They do this by interfering with chemical reactions within the body, downright *stealing* necessary vitamins and minerals from the body, and by creating an imbalance that throws all systems into a confounding quagmire.

So what are some of these imbalances that can wreak such havoc?

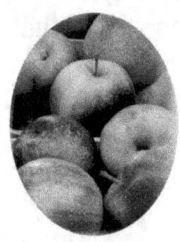

Chapter 1

The Omega 6 – Omega 3 Imbalance

The "Grand Imbalance" of Omega 6 and Omega 3 essential fatty acids is one of the most disruptive imbalances in the body. Not only is this imbalance a huge cause of inflammation, but it also causes cognitive issues, heart issues, hormonal issues, joint and cartilage issues, stomach issues, and lots more.

Why? Omega 6 is a pro-inflammatory (causes inflammation), and Omega 3 is an anti-inflammatory (helps fight inflammation). You can see where a balance of the two would be a GOOD thing here. If you are putting in a whole lot of inflammation-making foods, and *not* putting in an equal amount of *anti*-inflammatory foods, then it only stands to reason that you will reap the added inflammation!

We actually *need* both Omegas in our body. Both are *essential* fatty acids. In a perfect world, the Omega 6 helps the immune system by sending out warnings and inflammation to fight a cold or cut. This tells us that something is wrong and we must take care of it. The Omega 3 is an anti-inflammatory and healer, and balances this inflammation so that it doesn't take over. We deal with the cut or cold by taking aspirin; while the existing Omega 3 helps from the *inside* to ease pain and inflammation, so that things heal quickly. But this is in a perfect world. [1]

Omega 6

The problem is Omega 6 is everywhere, *far* outweighing Omega 3. Ideally these 6 and 3 Omegas should be balanced at 2:1 or 1:1. In actuality it is found to be 30:1 in some studies, and 50:1 in others! This is a LOT more inflammation than anti-inflammation. Is it any wonder that inflammatory autoimmune conditions have been so rampant in the past 50 years? [2]

Omega 6 is naturally found in healthy, real foods like nuts, beans and leafy greens, meats, poultry, eggs, grain & corn-fed animals, butter and cheese, and oils from corn, veggies, sunflower, safflower, canola, soybean, grape seed, canola, cotton seed, wheat germ, walnut and more—all healthy foods.

Note: Some herbs are *very* high in omega 6 – even in primrose oil, borage oil, and black cumin oil, e.g.

Secondary sources of omega 6's are prepared and

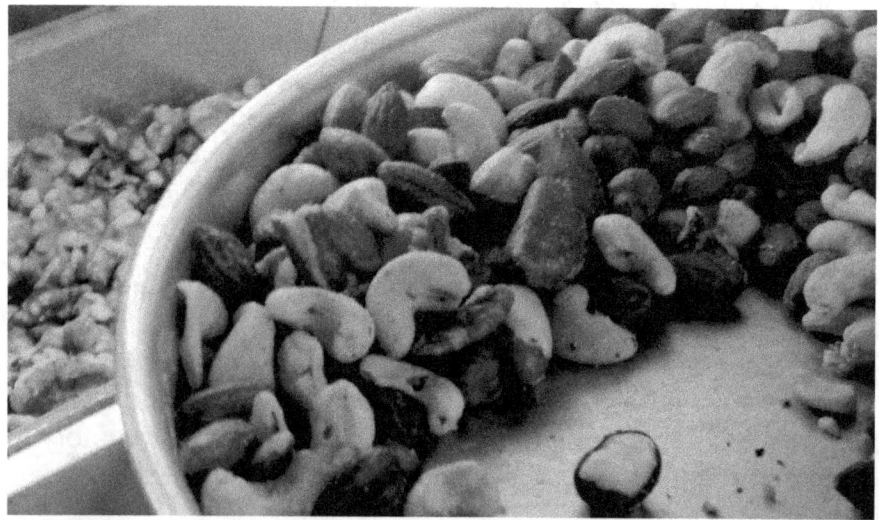

processed foods which utilize Omega 6's after they've been hydrogenated – items like margarines, mayonnaise, cooking oils, salad dressings, cereals, cookies, cakes, breads, whole grains, fried foods, etc.

The problem is that we not only eat the healthy foods with Omega 6—the grain-fed meats like eggs, butter, and leafy greens, but we also eat everything packaged and boxed with Omega 6's. These Omega 6 oils are only put into the products *after* they've been hydrogenated—to preserve shelf life, of course. The Omega 6 short-chain molecule is such a hardy little devil, it is next to impossible to cook or process it out, it just changes form – the form that makes even more inflammation in the form of hydrogenates or partially hydrogenates. *Jmyarlott.com* lists sources for Omega 6. It's everywhere! [3]

So where are the balancing anti-inflammatory Omega 3 fatty acids? They're found in fatty fish for the most part. How many folks eat fish every week? Not many. But I'd be willing to bet that *everyone* eats all the foods under the Omega 6 umbrella! Balance? Not hardly.

Omega 3 EPA-DHA

There are 3 kinds of Omega 3 fatty acids. Omega 3 EPA (eicosa pentaenoic acid), and DHA (docosa hexaenoic acid), are found in fish like salmon, sardines, mackerel, halibut, tuna, and in kelp, nori, algae, and sea vegetables. It is also found in grass-fed beef, venison, buffalo, wild turkey, free-range chicken, and their eggs – animals that have *never* eaten corn or grain (corn and grain are Omega 6's, which pretty much neutralize the animals' original Omega 3's).

Omega 3 EPA and DHA have been studied for many years at the National Institute of Health, the Mayo Clinic, and many medical universities for their treatment in heart conditions, high blood pressure, diabetes, rheumatoid arthritis, lupus, depression, osteoarthritis, Alzheimer's, ADHD, PTSD, cognitive issues, memory issues, Irritable Bowel Syndrome, macular degeneration, asthma, menstrual pain, mood swings, prostate and breast cancer, and more! [4]

There are *thousands* of studies where Omega 3 EPA-DHA has proven to help all these issues and more. This doesn't count all the many thousands (millions) of studies in the Netherlands, UK, Europe, and the Orient where they have been studying them since recorded history! They eat more fish than we do, and have for eons. [5]

According to Dr. William Sears, "DHA is the primary structural component of brain tissue, so it stands to reason that a deficiency of DHA in the diet could translate into a deficiency in brain function. In fact, research is increasingly recognizing the possibility that DHA has a crucial influence on neurotransmitters in the brain, helping brain cells better communicate with each other." [6]   Remember the only way we can get Omega 3 DHA is by eating foods with DHA or taking supplements. We have to go out and buy these foods and actually eat them on purpose, or intentionally take the supplements.

Omega 3 ALA

Omega 3 ALA (alpha linolenic acid) is the third anti-inflammatory Omega 3. This Omega 3 is found in plants like flax seed, walnuts, soybeans, and seeds. It's found in oils too, like soybean oil, flax seed oil, canola, sunflower & safflower oils, and most of the seed oils which also contain Omega 6. Some veggies also contain small amounts of Omega 3 ALA, such as Brussels sprouts, kale, spinach, and salad greens.

In healthy people, in a perfect world, this ALA Omega 3 short chain-fatty acid is partially converted in the body to small amounts of Omega 3 EPA-DHA long-chain fatty acids, the type that does the heavy duty work and healing. This conversion is not really dependable though, especially in those with a chronic illness. According to The University of Maryland Medical

Center, "ALA from flax and other vegetarian sources needs to be converted in the body to EPA and DHA. Many people do not make these conversions very effectively, however." [7]

This is not to say that Omega 3 ALA is not helpful. Quite the contrary; it is also an anti-inflammatory and has been found to be good for many health issues. In fact, vegetarians often rely on this ALA form of Omega 3. [8] The benefits are not quite the same as the EPA-DHA, however. I would therefore recommend adding kelp, nori, algae, or other sea vegetables to obtain sufficient DHA to the vegetarian diet. [9] In other words Omega 3 ALA should not be used as a substitute for Omega 3 EPA-DHA, but rather in addition to them.

An important note here: It's true that Omega 6 and 3 are *both* found in many of the above described seed oils and veggies; however, after cooking or processing, only the Omega 6 will remain. This is because the short-chained Omega 6 molecule is a hardy little devil and can withstand high heat (500-1000°) for several hours and come up smelling like a hydrogenated rose, whereas the Omega 3 becomes oxidized and completely neutralized as anything beneficial with heat over 120°.

Unfortunately, the short chain Omega 3 ALA molecules (like the long-chain Omega 3 EPA-DHA) are quite delicate and fragile. Temperatures over 120° begins oxidizing them and soon renders them null…but not void. After being oxidized they are no longer of value to anyone's body. This oxidized Omega 3 oil is no longer recognizable as a healthy fat, and it will now, literally, *put* free radicals into your body by the bucketsful with every bite! Inflammation comes with these free radicals—for free, of course! Light and air also oxidize this fragile molecule. So once the walnut, soybean, or Brussels sprout is opened or cut and exposed to air and light (or cooked), the good Omega 3 begins oxidizing, whereas the Omega 6 will stand strong as the pro-inflammatory that it is. Like an apple after being cut, the oxidation process begins immediately. [10]

Omega 3's are Fats

For those who are shaking their heads saying, "But we're supposed to eat a low-fat diet!" I say, "Au Contraire!" Excess animal saturated fats, hydrogenated fats, and trans fats are the fats that were used in those tests so many years ago. But no one bothered to mention that detail. Indeed, these are the fats to avoid like a cow patty! The trouble is, "the-powers-that-be" lumped all fats together and said, simply, "No fats." This was a huge dis-service to the American people.

According to the Harvard School of Public Health, in the 1960s when [mostly healthy] fats and oils supplied 45% of the American diet, about 13% of Americans were obese and 1% had type 2 diabetes. Then in the 80s when we were told to stop eating fats and began eating a low fat diet, we progressively became less healthy, and today 33% of our diet consists of fats [mostly hydrogenated now], and 34% of our adult population is obese and 11% have type 2 diabetes! This does not even include the rising percentage of our children who are obese! [11]

Healthy fats are absolutely necessary to the human body! They provide healthy cell membranes for efficient nutritional transfer; they enable our hormones to function efficiently; they "feed" our brain; they enable our neurons to fire and cells to communicate with each other; they lubricate our joints, tendons and ligaments; they keep the myelin sheath (surrounding our muscles and organs) supple and malleable; they enable the absorption of fat soluble vitamins like A, D, E, and K (they cannot *be* absorbed without fats); they are a valuable source of energy; they prevent dry hair, dry skin, dry eye, and so much more. Fats? We *have* to *have* them! Many of our issues may be a case of the missing fats – GOOD fats! [12]

TIP So do we kill all the Omega 3's when cooking our salmon and grass-fed beef? No. When cooking gently at a medium to low temperature, the outside of the salmon or beef steak is seared and oxidized, sealing in all the good Omega 3's, while the inside is cooking slowly, and at a lower temperature. It's when it's cooked to death at a high temp, through and through that the interior Omega 3's are destroyed. An oxidized apple, for example, can still be eaten after the serious oxidation is scraped off; the apple is still filled with thousands of beneficial nutrients. Nutrients that in fact help neutralize that oxidation!

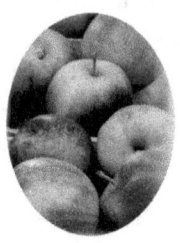

Chapter 2

The Calcium - Magnesium Imbalance

Carolyn Dean, MD, ND, author of *The Magnesium Miracle* (Ballentine 2007), and 30 other books on magnesium and health, states that the action of calcium is pro-inflammatory, while that of magnesium is anti-inflammatory. She also tells us that excess calcium can and does create a magnesium deficiency.[1]

That seems to be where most all of us are at the moment, especially if we have an autoimmune illness. Along with the excess calcium in our bodies, is the deficiency of magnesium to further complicate the issue. Any magnesium that *is* introduced (eaten) is used up by a chronically ill body at warp speed!

This surprising imbalance is becoming more and more recognized, thank goodness. Well, that's not exactly accurate. I should say that many doctors are finally paying attention to the studies – a study called The Harvard Nurses Study, in particular. We are indeed under a cloud of excess calcium and magnesium insufficiency!

The Harvard Nurses Study took place between 1980 and 1992, and followed 77,761 women ages 34 to 59. They wanted to find out if there was a relationship between milk consumption and osteoporosis. They were concerned because, although Americans drink more milk than any other country in the world, we also have the *highest* incidence of osteoporosis, bone disease and bone fracture! What was that? The most milk drinkers AND the most bone disease?

We know that calcium supplementation doesn't do any better for us either! Calcium supplements have been recommended by doctors for 50 years, and bone disease, osteopenia, osteoporosis, and bone fracture is at an all-time high! [2]

Yet, a study in China, soon after the Harvard study, found that people in small outer provinces who drank NO milk, ever, had never *heard* of bone disease or osteoporosis. How can that be? [3]

The China Study (BenBella Books, 2006), by Dr. T. Colin Campbell explains in detail about this study, and information about our American diet in general. Indeed, it is the most comprehensive study of health and nutrition ever conducted. I highly recommend it for in-depth reading. But I digress.

Earl Staelin, a medical researcher and attorney well-known for defending his clients rights to alternative care, has written a remarkable three-part series titled "Strong Bones or Osteoporosis" for the March/April 2006 issue of the *Well Being Journal* (back issues are available at wellbeingjournal. com), in which he explains how excess calcium and insufficient magnesium can cause so much pain.[4] He cites specific examples of "miraculous" cures simply by *decreasing* calcium intake to half the (RDA) Recommended Daily Allowance and *increasing* magnesium intake to a ratio closer to one-to-one with calcium. Further, he states, "…high calcium consumption may actually interfere with calcium absorption, resulting in weaker bones, and cause calcium to be deposited where it is not wanted!" This of course refers to potential bone spurs, kidney stones, calcium deposits in breast tissue, organs, and joints.

Dr. Phillip Rosenblum, medical director and president of Arbor Family Medicine in Bloomfield, CO, wrote an article in the July/August 2006 issue of the *Well Being Journal*, titled "Calcium, Magnesium, and Horsetail Supplementation," stating that he [and every other medical student, whether at Harvard, Yale or other] had no formal training in vitamins, minerals, and supplements. He goes on to say, "I began to become convinced that calcium supplements were not the benign supplements I had assumed, but rather were actually causing actual physical harm and discomfort."

He describes several cases in which his patients had "suddenly" become much better—a few in particular were greatly helped, after 25 years of suffering, when their calcium intake was lowered and magnesium intake summarily rose. When treating fibromyalgia patients, he says, "I am becoming convinced that the spectre of fibromyalgia can be largely explained by calcium excess and/or magnesium deficiency."

Excess is the issue here. Excess calcium. It's true, calcium is the most prevalent mineral in the body, and ninety-nine percent of it is stored in the body as bones and teeth. Yet, *all of it* works in partnership with magnesium in a sort of "push-pull" manner. Calcium contracts; magnesium relaxes. Nearly everything calcium does in the body is balanced by the alternate reaction of magnesium. [5]

Calcium uses magnesium to absorb and to perform the "push-pull" thing. Yet, when you buy a supplement that contains both minerals, and a multi-vitamin, you'll find the ratio of calcium to magnesium is 3 or 4:1. [6]

So what happens is that calcium uses up *all* the magnesium just to get absorbed, leaving no magnesium for the all-important 325+ functions that magnesium is responsible for. In fact, the leftover calcium still requires magnesium to get its remaining molecules absorbed, and so it then robs the magnesium it needs from muscle, blood, bone, and so on. Then, if there is *still* calcium left over, it may leave via urine, OR it may sit in a cell, unable to go anywhere or do anything because there's no magnesium around.

This extra calcium molecule has contracted the cell and it sits there, tapping its foot, waiting for a magnesium molecule to come along to relax the cell. But with all this extra calcium floating around, it's much simpler to combine with another calcium molecule…then another and another and so on. With all these other calcium molecules, the cell soon becomes calcified and unusable, killing the cell. This calcified clump then accumulates with other cells of its kind and, bingo…you have PAIN. It shows up in the form of an unwanted calcium deposit latching onto muscle, organs, the brain, joints (e.g. bone spur), or elsewhere. When calcium is not fully utilized, by equal amounts of magnesium, this under-absorption can lead to all sorts of problems. [7]

A number of studies [PubMed abstracts #9641824, 2133625, 3199134, and many others indexed for Medline] have shown that taking magnesium lactate or intravenous magnesium sulfate (both readily absorbable forms of magnesium, as is magnesium malate, aspartate, and glycinate) will effectively break up those calcification deposits and greatly help the pain caused by them. [8]

Topically applied magnesium, in the form of magnesium chloride, whether in an oil spray or gel form, flakes or salts, e.g. Epsom salts, is also immediately helpful and also very well-absorbed. Topical magnesium doesn't go through the digestive system; it is absorbed into the skin, where it goes directly into muscles and then into your bloodstream where it is transported to everywhere else it's needed. Soaking for 20 minutes in a hot bath of Epsom salts is…priceless! Or spraying magnesium oil onto your muscles or the soles of your feet at bedtime is just as effective. Magnesium oil or salts are quite well-absorbed through the skin…and quite effective in helping many kinds of pain. [9]

***

"There is no substitute for magnesium; it's as close as a metal comes to being as necessary as air."

~Mark Sircus Ac., OMD

Mark Sircus Ac., OMD states, "There has been a steep decline of dietary magnesium in the United States, from a high of almost 500 mg/day at the turn of the last century to barely 175-225 mg/day today. The National Academy of Sciences has determined that most Americans are magnesium deficient, with men obtaining only about 80 percent of their daily needs with women fairing even worse obtaining about 70 percent of their needs." Not surprisingly, these percentages are pertaining to healthy people. I suspect for those who are suffering a chronic illness (or two) these numbers are markedly lower.

Dr. Jerry Aikawa, from the University of Colorado, author of, "Magnesium: Its Biological Significance," states, "Magnesium is the most important mineral to man and all living organisms." In fact, he states, "Without magnesium, muscle and nerve functions are compromised and energy diminished. We are operating with the power turned off." [10]

So what causes this *deficiency* in magnesium? Excess calcium, for one. But, if you enjoy soda pop, alcoholic drinks, nicotine, coffee, processed meats like hot dogs or bologna, starches and carbohydrates, such as items made with white flour, white sugar, high fructose corn syrup, or salty foods, your magnesium stores are being eaten up with every bite. These foods actually increase your *need* for magnesium. Food processing literally removes magnesium from foods, as does frying, broiling, steaming, and boiling. Some of these processed foods, however, can cause your existing magnesium to become unusable by binding it in the gut to create magnesium phosphate, a salt that cannot be used in the body, and is subsequently released in the urine. In essence, these foods are *"stealing your magnesium."* This is *not* a good thing. [11]

Prolonged stress, emotional and physical, also leads to magnesium deficiencies. Even loud noises or sleep deprivation can cause magnesium loss. If your body is trying to repair damaged tissue, e.g. arthritis or bone fracture, your magnesium is being used up like crazy. Older adults are more likely to have low levels of magnesium. People with low calcium or potassium levels usually have magnesium deficiency as well. Then, of course, if you are subject to profuse sweating, irritable bowel syndrome, Crohn's disease, *hyper*thyroidism, diabetes, kidney malfunction, heart disease, gluten intolerance, heavy menstrual periods, dietary or digestion problems, or if you suffer from vomiting or diarrhea during a flu episode, your magnesium absorption capability becomes extremely limited. [12]

Deficiencies can also occur because your body simply can't absorb a significant amount of magnesium through the regular channels. There are asthma medications, diuretics, birth control pills, corticosteroids, antibiotics and other prescription drugs that can cause magnesium to become blocked or unusable and lost in urine. If this magnesium is not being replenished, it is actually adding *more* pain to the existing issue! [13]

Fibromyalgia, for example, with its muscle aches, exhaustion, emotional and physical stress, lack of sleep, IBS, digestion problems, and all the other potential symptoms can *not only* deplete magnesium, but can also be the *result* of depleted magnesium. It's another one of those chicken and egg conundrums. [14]

There is a mnemonic that medical students use to remember some of *the effects of excessive calcium (which means by default, deficient magnesium)*: "**Groans, Moans, Bones, Stones, and Psychiatric Overtones**." Meaning: constipation, body aches, fragile bone pain, kidney stones, mental confusion and depression. Other signs and symptoms include fatigue, depression, nausea, and more. Of course,

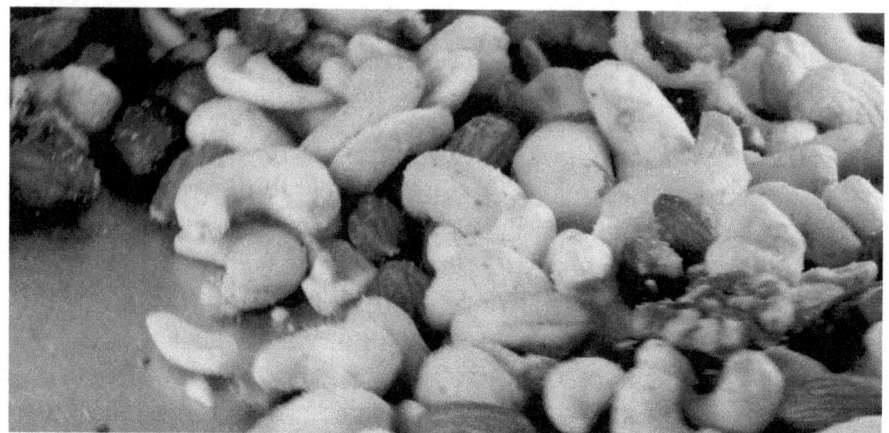

stress has a lot to do with these listed conditions, but then stress "steals" magnesium, no matter what your condition, leaving calcium the only game in town. Groans, moans, bones, stones, & psychiatric overtones, indeed!

Balance is the thing. The moral of this story is to try your own little test to see if you can help relieve some of your pain by temporarily stopping the calcium supplements and cutting back on calcium foods for a week or so, and then *add* more magnesium foods. Milk, cheese, yogurt, and other dairy products are full of calcium, but there are many other foods containing calcium too.

The *Agricultural Research Service (ARS) Nutrient Database* website provides a list of foods rich in calcium that are non-dairy. [15] They include foods such as: sardines, tofu, salmon, collard greens, spinach, oatmeal, white beans, kale, beet greens, dandelion greens, and more. In addition, the *National Institutes of Health* website provides a huge shopping list of magnesium rich foods; it includes foods such as almonds, spinach, oatmeal, Brazil nuts, almonds, cashews, peanuts, peanut butter, baked potato with skin, brown rice, lentils, chocolate and much more. [16] Or you can use a search engine and type in "foods with calcium" and "foods with magnesium" to get a head start.

The idea here is to stop eating and drinking foods that deplete your magnesium. In other words, allow the magnesium to catch up with the excess calcium; and after that, maintain a magnesium/calcium balance closer to 1:1.

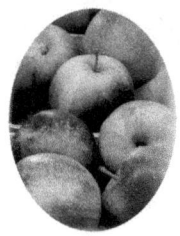

Chapter 3

The Acid – Alkaline Imbalance

The acid-alkaline measurement of all things fluid, including the fluids in your body, is measured in pH (potential of Hydrogen). A low or high reading here is not so much a "condition" as a very important *indicator* of things to come. Much like a see-saw this balancing scale is "0," at the most acidic, exemplified by sulfuric acid (powerful stuff) and "14," at the most alkaline, where chalk resides. Either endpoint is deadly for a human body. The pivot point, "7," is neutral, and pure water is the ideal example.

Sulfuric acid	*Water*	*Chalk*
0	7	14

Fig. 1

Pati Chandler

This scale is not a simple "1, 2, 3" scale however; the pH values are logarithmic. To make a long story short, a pH of 6 is actually 10 times more acidic than 7. A pH of 5 is *100* times more acidic; 4 is 1,000 times more acidic and a pH of 3 is *10,000* times more acidic than the neutral 7, and so on. So when you learn that soft drinks are 2.3 to 3.0 on this pH scale you will understand that your soft drink is at least 10,000 times *more acidic* than water, and much closer to sulfuric acid than you ever want to be!

The Body's Normal pH

The human body, especially the blood, spinal fluid and saliva, is 7.4 on this pH scale. This means that our body generally needs to be slightly alkaline in nature. But nothing within the body is static; there are constant fluctuations and adjustments even in the healthiest body all day long. This pH varies within a narrow window of 7.36 to 7.45 depending on the time of day, the food you eat, the amount of stress you are dealing with, the amount of sleep you get, whether you are fighting an infection or have a chronic illness and so on.

The pH of the body's fluids is also work-specific. That is, different areas of your body will have a different pH. The digestive system, for example, must maintain an acidic pH in order to digest food. Your skin must remain slightly acidic to fight off the everyday germs and bacteria it comes in contact with. Urine is more acidic because its job is to release acids and toxins. Enzymes and proteins must stay within a specific narrow acidic range in order to get their jobs done and etc.

However, things can get out of hand in a hurry when an alkaline area, such as the blood, strays outside its designated pH boundary and dips too far to the acidic side. Fortunately, your body can automatically tip the scales back to adjust its own pH. It does this by taking the alkaline minerals it needs from the calcium storehouses such as bones and teeth, in order to help re-balance this pH and bring it back to the desired alkaline state. This is called *homeostasis*.

Note: Homeostasis is responsible for regulating many internal functions—blood pressure, temperature, electrolytes, and much more.

Homeostasis is the body's activity of regulating its own internal environment and working at maintaining a stable, constant condition. [1]

Under certain circumstances, however, this mechanism doesn't work efficiently for some reason, or in the case of your body's pH, the quantity of the acids far exceeds the level at which it can be managed.

The more stress, the more erratic sleep, the more acid-forming *foods and drinks* you consume, the more your body teeters toward the acidic. The more your body leans to the acidic, the more alkalinizing minerals (calcium, magnesium, potassium and sodium) your body will take (or steal) from bones, teeth, organs, and even blood in order to save itself.

This act in itself creates even more stress on your body. This goes way beyond the normal, gentle balancing act of homeostasis. Dr. Susan E. Brown and Larry Trivieri co-authored *The Acid Alkaline Food Guide* (Square One Publishers, 2006), an excellent short guide to how foods affect the pH balance in our bodies, which describes this process quite well. In a Natural News.com article, "The Acid-Alkaline Food Guide: Interview with the Author," Dr. Phil Domenico conducted a very informative interview with Larry Trivieri about the book. [2]

A body with a chronic illness is already on the acidic side. The idea here is to stop pushing down on this side of the scale! If your body is already robbing Peter to pay Paul by taking alkalinizing minerals from wherever it can just to maintain this balance due to your illness, it only stands to reason that you wouldn't want to add to the acidic condition by filling it full of acidic foods!

Virtually *all* degenerative diseases, including cancer, heart disease, osteoporosis, arthritis, and more are associated with excess acidity in the body. These diseases literally *thrive* in an acidic atmosphere, and cannot survive in an alkaline atmosphere! Stress alone has been described as "eating away at your insides." [3, 4]

Note: Cognitive Behavioral Therapy (CBT), deep breathing, prayer, meditation, EFT, Yoga, and Tai Chi are just a few excellent ways to de-stress *and* de-acidify!

This Balance is 25/75

In the meantime, cutting back on acid-forming foods, and adding more alkalinizing foods will help immeasurably. However, it's not possible, nor even advisable, to stop eating acid-forming foods all together. It's also not advisable to eat *only* alkalinizing foods. It's all about BALANCE! [5]

The proper balance of acidic to alkaline is 25% acidic and 75% alkaline. Sometimes we unconsciously *try* to balance things, thinking that one balances the other. For example, bacon goes with eggs, meat goes with potatoes, coffee goes with cream, cereal goes with milk, and perhaps making a cheese sandwich with wheat bread. In actuality, *all* of these are acidic or acid-forming foods, making the percentages severely skewed to the acidic. [6] These typical examples contain no alkaline foods at all – no fruits and veggies, nearly all of which are alkaline - and nowhere near 75% alkaline of the meal. It is quite the reverse, in fact.

When there is a glut of acidic foods and/or drinks, without the proper balance of alkaline, we run into homeostatic problems where the quantities of acids exceeds the body's ability to continuously and successfully manage it. For example, to neutralize, or to balance the acid in one can of soda (2.5 pH), you would need to drink 32 eight oz. glasses of alkaline water (pH 7.5-8). So you can see how one can of cola starts the day off at a major deficit, and your body begins robbing Peter to pay Paul! [7]

To achieve a successful balancing act, one must look at whether a certain food or drink is acid-forming or alkaline-forming rather than whether it is strictly an acid or alkaline food in and of itself. Citrus fruits, like lemons and limes, are by themselves acidic foods. However, once these foods are inside the body, they are converted to bicarbonates—alkaline chemicals. So putting a slice of lemon or lime in your water or tea is a GOOD thing! Apple Cider Vinegar (ACV) is the same – acidic by itself, but when you put 1-2 tsp. into a glass of water and drink, it turns into an alkaline-forming drink, helping your body immeasurably! And of course drinking bicarbonate of soda (baking soda) – 1-2 tsp. in a glass of water – is a definite alkalizer. An excellent book on finding out more about acid/alkaline foods and suggestions on how to maintain that balance is *The Acid Alkaline Food Guide* by Dr. Susan E. Brown and Larry Trivieri as mentioned above.

You can probably guess what some acid-forming foods are. The prime acid-forming foods are sugar (and all its aliases), artificial sweeteners, soft drinks, and simple carbohydrates. Also, meats, white rice, whole grains, cheese, many nuts, some seeds, alcoholic drinks, mustard, ketchup, mayonnaise, and many more, along with tobacco, are all acid-forming when consumed. [8]

It's interesting to note that Sucanat (evaporated cane juice), coconut sugar and *raw unpasteurized* honey are alkaline. A sugar substitute made from chicory root called *Just Like Sugar*® (available at *Amazon.com*) is also alkaline with a pH of 8. Practically all fruits and veggies are alkaline, as well as freshly squeezed fruit juices, all freshly-squeezed vegetable juices, garlic, most herbs and herbal teas, most spices, and of course, sodium bicarbonate (Arm & Hammer® Baking Soda, e.g.) are all alkaline.

The idea is not to eliminate acids *or* to overload on alkalines, but rather to aim at the 25% to 75% acid-alkaline balance to help your body maintain things at a happy 7.4 pH. To find out more about pH in the body or for a full list of acid-forming and alkaline-forming foods, check Rense.com [9] or *The Acid Alkaline Food Guide* mentioned above.

TIP ONE   Bottled drinking water can also be acid or alkaline. Distilled water and Reverse Osmosis water are waters that have had minerals filtered out (deleted) and have a pH of 4 - 4.5. It is the calcium, magnesium, potassium and sodium, and minerals which make the water alkaline. Some of the most popular bottled waters have a similar pH of 4. Chlorinated water (tap water) is mostly acid-forming with a pH below 7, depending on how much chlorine is in it. You would do well to add pH balancing drops such as Body Rescue®, Cell Food®, Alka Max Alkaline Booster®, True Alka™ or some similar alkaline additive drops. [10] These are mineral drops in a liquid form that can be added to your bottle of water to raise the pH level. *Or* you can add lime, lemon, or Apple Cider Vinegar as mentioned above. Another option is adding 1-2 tsp. of bicarbonate soda to your bottled water. You can test the pH of the water or any bottled waters in your home with pH test strips available at any pet store where they sell aquariums and/or pet fish. You can also use diabetic test strips. Remember, you are aiming at finding water with a minimum pH of 7.0 (neutral), preferably 8.0 or more.

TIP TWO   Some good pH + bottled drinking waters are: Fiji®, Icelandic Spring®, Evian®, Arrowhead®, Crystal Geyser®, Deep Park®, Deep Rock®, Evamore®, Ice Mountain®, Volvic®, Penta®, and natural spring waters (with a high mineral content) or mineral water. [11]   If you want to know the pH of any specific bottled water, you can also call the company that bottles it and ask what the pH is. Please be kind to your eco system and get the large gallon bottles and pour it into your stainless steel drinking bottle. There are so many small plastic bottles now we will soon be buried in them!

Is There a Diet for Chronic Illness?

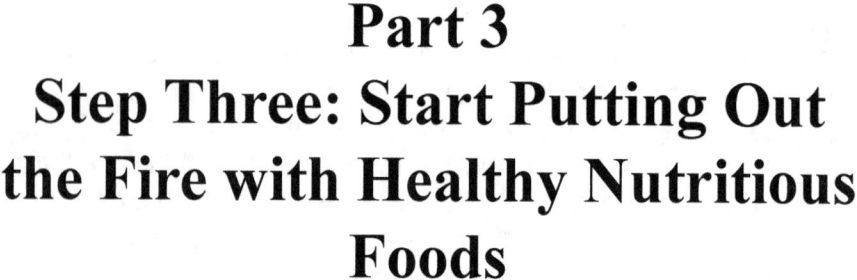

Part 3
Step Three: Start Putting Out the Fire with Healthy Nutritious Foods

"Let food be your medicine and medicine be your food."

~Hippocrates

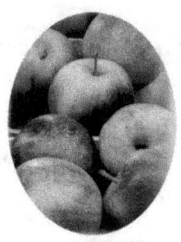

Chapter 1

The Relationship between Food and Pain

You are *not* powerless in controlling your pain and symptoms. You actually have the advantage! Indeed, you have a much *better* means at your disposal than anyone in the medical field. You can choose what you eat and drink; and, your choices can make a *huge* difference.

We know that our body needs certain kinds of fuel in order to operate at peak efficiency—namely proteins, fats, and carbohydrates. These basic three contain all the amino acids, saturated fats, polyunsaturated fats, monounsaturated fats, vitamins, minerals, fiber, starch, enzymes, probiotics and prebiotics, etc. that our body requires to work at peak efficiency. All the nutrients in these basic three promote growth, maintenance and *repair* of our body on a daily basis.

Anything that *does not* promote growth, maintenance and repair is unnecessary and may likely cause a reverse in this process, leading or adding to chronic illnesses. Some prime examples of these can be found in Part 1.

Proteins, fats, and carbohydrates supply all the essentials that are needed to regulate our systems – hormonal, cardiovascular, pulmonary, lymphatic, sensory, nervous,

> *You are not powerless in
> controlling your pain and symptoms.
> You can choose what you eat and drink;
> and your choices can make a huge
> difference in your pain!*

muscular, skeletal, and all the rest. They provide the proper fuel to enable our body to grow, maintain and repair itself in the course of a normal day. For those with a chronic illness, these basic three are not just "nice to have," they are essential; indeed they are *crucial*!

Note: You can forget the idea that fats are evil. They are in fact as necessary as oxygen! You just need the *right kinds* of fats.

A chronically ill body uses up much of its resources just to fight the illness. And when a body is weak from this daily fight, it has the near impossible job of just trying to "catch up" to normal. As important as it is to eliminate the foods and drinks that cause inflammation and add to our pain, it is also crucial to give your body the nutrition it needs to function at its peak efficiency every single day.

The Word "Diet"

When one hears the word "diet" the first thing that comes to mind is the thought of giving up foods in order to lose weight. The concept in this book has more to do with a "way of eating" for health. Rather than giving up foods, my focus is more on what to eat and why; and by extension, what *not* to eat and why.

> *The focus is on what to eat
> for your health and why.*

Pati Chandler

Although many with chronic illnesses have an issue with weight, either excess or not enough, the diets listed below can and do lead to a healthy body, and may indeed affect weight issues at the same time.

Please keep in mind, however, that choosing a method of eating for weight control alone is not in our best interests. We who are chronically ill need to eat healthy, non-inflammatory foods in order to maintain a body that can heal itself effectively and not interfere with any supplements or medications that are necessary for our specific illness. "Fake" foods, inflammatory foods, and foods that have zero nutrition interfere with the very purpose of our body. The human body was made to heal itself, which it can and does do when fed the proper nutrients. It cannot heal itself when stuffed with plastic and imitation foods with no nutritional value.

Diets for Health

There are any number of temporary fad diets – the cabbage diet, the grapefruit diet, the low fat diet, the low carb diet, etc. Then there are the DASH Diet, the South Beach Diet®, Atkins Diet, The Zone® Diet, The TLC Diet, Weight Watchers®, Jenny Craig®, Nutrisystem®, Vegetarian, Vegan and so on. [1] In fact, *The US News* has listed and rated 29 diets on their Health & Wellness webpage. Most of these are geared towards losing weight.

> *What I am sharing here are beneficial foods for your health—a life-healthy way of eating.*

The three healthiest ways of eating are the following three "diets." However, finding your own balance and your own "system" is key to what works best for you. You may want to

Is There a Diet for Chronic Illness?

incorporate parts of each of these three or do something even a bit differently. Whatever way of eating you choose, keeping inflammation at bay, keeping the balance and putting out the fire are essential. Each of these three diets accomplishes these goals.

1) **Mediterranean Diet.** According to the Mayo Clinic, the Mediterranean Diet in general is classified as one of the healthiest ways of eating. [2]

   The Mediterranean diet emphasizes:

   - Eating primarily plant-based foods – fruits, veggies, whole grains, legumes, nuts

   - Replacing butter with healthy fats, such as olive oil

   - Using herbs and spices, instead of salt to flavor foods

   - Limiting red meat to no more than a few times a month

   - Eating fish and poultry at least twice a week

   - Drinking red wine in moderation (optional)

2) **Caveman Diet.**

   The Caveman Diet emphasizes:

   - High protein intake

   - Lower carbohydrate intake and lower glycemic index

   - High fiber intake

   - Moderate to higher fat intake dominated by

monounsaturated and polyunsaturated fats with balanced Omega-3 and Omega-6 fats

- High potassium, lower sodium intake

- A general balance of acid/alkaline intake

- Higher intake of, vitamins, minerals, antioxidants, and plant phytochemicals [3]

3) Food Combining Diet. A lesser known, though much older way of eating involves combining your foods in a healthy way. Ayurvedic Medicine and even the Jewish kashrut laws had found that food combining was indeed the healthiest way to eat thousands of years ago. [4]

The Food Combining diet emphasizes three basic rules:

- Never combine proteins and starchy carbohydrates at a meal

- Never combine fruits and veggies, or fruits and protein at a meal

- Always eat fruits alone, between meals

There are many neutral foods that can be eaten with the carb meal or the protein meal – lettuce, uncooked tomato, lentils, yogurt, cottage cheese, nuts, and more. Some foods considered proteins and others considered carbs in this diet may surprise you, however. The foods are considered by nutrient, not by food category. It can get a bit complicated. For a list of foods considered protein and carbohydrates and a full list of neutral foods I recommend a visit to the *Food Combining*

Diet's website. [5]

Jane Lear, former editor of *Gourmet,* current blogger, and author explains the "science" behind the reasoning of food combining:

> …The reasoning is as follows: Since protein digestion utilizes enzymes that are more acidic than the ones utilized by carbs, when you eat those two types of foods at once, the enzymes cancel each other out, thus the food can't be assimilated. Instead, it sits in your system and rots or ferments, building up as toxic material in your colon… [6]

This often creates gas, bloating, intestinal discomfort, and

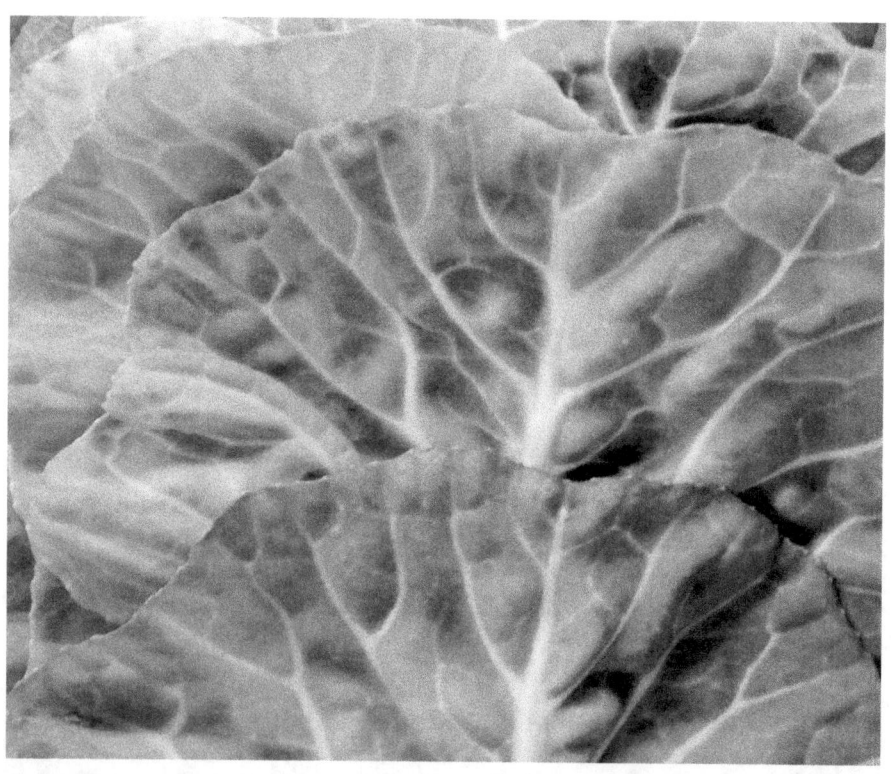

incomplete digestion. Similar activity occurs when fruits and veggies are eaten together; the enzymes required to digest each, cancel each other out. Fruits are digested at warp speed because of the high sugar content. So, eating them alone and on an empty stomach about 1.5 to 2 hours before your next meal is the way to go here. This provides instant useable glucose—energy.

There are benefits to each of these ways of eating. And each "diet" does best with eliminating inflammatory foods and balancing minerals, fatty acids and acid/alkaline foods, while adding LOTS of good anti-inflammatory foods to put out the fire! Because not everything works for everyone, just as being a vegan or eating a protein diet is not for everyone, you must test and try it in order to choose what works best for your body.

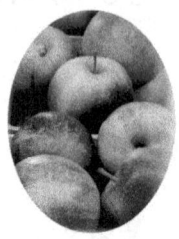

Chapter 2

Those Important "Little Things"

Our gut has been called the "Second Brain" for good reason. Michael Gershon, Chairman of the Department of Anatomy and Cell Biology at the New York-Presbyterian Hospital/Columbia University Medical Center, is the author of *The Second Brain* (HarperCollins, 1998). Here, he describes the enteric nervous system, which consists of sheaths of neurons embedded into the nine meters of our alimentary canal (from end to end), totaling more than 100 million neurons – more than in the spinal cord or the peripheral nervous system.

These neurons are responsible for more than just digestion. Do you ever get "butterflies" in your stomach when you're nervous? Or do you get that "gut-wrenching" feeling when something goes terribly wrong? Researchers have discovered that 90% of the fibers in the vagus nerve send signals *from* the gut *to* the brain, not the other way around. This enteric nervous system in the gut uses more than 30 neurotransmitters. In fact, 95% of the body's neurotransmitter, serotonin, is found in the bowels!

This relatively new field of study called neurogastroenterology is finding major connections between the gut and autoimmune diseases. Only recently, researchers have discovered a possible connection between the leaking of serotonin from the gut to play a part in autism. [1]

Natasha Campbell-McBride, MD, author of *Gut and Psychology Syndrome* (GAPS). *Natural Treatment for Autism, ADHD/ADD, Dyslexia, Dyspraxia, Depression and Schizophrenia* (Medinform Publishing, 2010) has designed a self-help program for treating disease through diet. The GAPS nutritional protocol helps to heal allergies, Chronic Fatigue Syndrome, fibromyalgia, Adrenal Fatigue, and many more. [2]

"All diseases begin in the gut." This is not a new concept. Hippocrates was the first to voice this statement more than a thousand years ago. We really *are* what we eat. So you can see where the care and feeding of our gut is critical.

Everyone knows that we need vitamins and minerals of course, and those little incidentals like oxygen and water. But what about those important "little things," like enzymes, probiotics and prebiotics that focus their attention in the gut? These are the very "little things" that enable, not only the proper breakdown and digestion of proteins, fats and carbohydrates, but enable your body to function at its peak efficiency.

For those with sensitive stomachs or intestinal issues like IBS, IBD, Crohn's, etc, these may be the most important of all for proper digestion and ease of symptoms. Yet, enzymes do much more than just help your body breakdown food so it can be absorbed. We also need them for all of our metabolic functions. Without enzymes, we are in serious trouble! According to Humbart Santillo, ND, "No chemical action or reaction can take place in the body without enzymes!" [2a]

Enzymes

More than three thousand enzymes have been identified, and researchers suspect there may be upwards of 50,000 enzymes in total.

Enzymes are enablers; they make it possible for biological reactions to take place. One enzyme works with phosphorous to build bone; another helps digest one particular kind of protein; still another will help coagulate blood when you get a cut; another helps eliminate carbon dioxide from your lungs when you breathe; others help in the construction of new muscle, nerve or skin tissues; others help the liver, kidney, lung, and skin in removing waste from the body; others work to help breakdown and digest some fat, or a particular milk-sugar or carbohydrate and so on.

Enzymes are involved in literally every biological function in our body. They are catalysts made up of amino acids, and each enzyme has one specific function that no other enzyme can do. [3] So you can see where you would need *all* possible enzymes daily.

We are actually born with all the enzymes we need. Isn't that nice? However, Dr. Joseph Mercola tells us, "Studies show that, every ten years, your body's production of enzymes [mostly produced by the pancreas] decreases by 13 percent. So by age 40, your enzyme production could be 25 percent lower than when you were a child. And by the time you're 70 you could be producing only ONE-THIRD of the enzymes you need."

Note: This is a description of a typical, "ideal" situation for a *healthy* person. [4]

Our lifestyle can diminish our stores of enzymes, too. Our body's enzymes are destroyed by alcohol consumption, caffeine, cigarette smoke, fluoridated water, stress, acidic foods and drinks, prescription drugs, pesticides, free radicals, ultra-violet radiation, x-rays, and much more. And the enzymes found in food are destroyed by heat over 118 degrees, so if you are trying to acquire enzymes by eating fresh foods, any major cooking is out. [5]

As you get older and your pancreas begins naturally

slowing down on the job, your body will pull the enzymes it needs from your stores in the liver, spleen, kidney, heart, lungs etc. This of course means consequences for these organs. Enzymes can be "lost" too, rather than just used up. Dr. Santillo tells us that "...many tests have shown that various enzymes are found in urine after the heat of fevers and athletic activity. We lose enzymes every day through our sweat, urine, feces, and all digestive fluids, including salivary and intestinal secretions." [5a]

What this means is that we must add them daily. We do this by eating raw, ideally organic foods which contain enzymes and, if necessary, by taking enzyme supplements. This not only adds enzymes to help us digest food and maintain our metabolic functions, but it boosts our body's ability to make more of its own enzymes.[6]

Some of our body's own enzymes like, superoxide dismutase (SOD), glutathione peroxidase (GPO) and catalase (CAT) for example, are also exceptionally important *antioxidants*. Proteolytic enzymes (protein enzymes, or proteases) such as bromelain, papain, etc. that we get from foods, aid in digesting proteins, but they are also excellent *anti-inflammatories*. Other enzymes use certain minerals and vitamins to help in their work. These are called CO-enzymes, the most famous of which is Co-enzyme Q10, or CoQ10, noted as a super antioxidant for the heart. But, CoQ10's most important role is in the mitochondria of each cell in your body, where it helps to make energy, in the form of that all-important ATP molecule (adenosine triphosphate) – our cell's very life energy!

Magnesium assists in this ATP energy-making process with CoQ10, and in over 325 other enzyme reactions. This is why it is imperative to have a sufficient amount of magnesium in our body. These reactions don't happen without the proper fuel!

There are three classes of enzymes:

1. Digestive enzymes that are produced in the body to aid in digestion.

2. Metabolic enzymes that work in the body's blood, tissues, and organs.

3. Food enzymes that are contained in *raw* food, which aid both of the above.

Digestive Enzymes

The digestive process starts in your mouth, or more specifically in your saliva. As you chew your food, breaking it down into smaller mashed up bits, the enzymes in your saliva begin the process of digestion. Your saliva's enzymes continue working all the way down to the stomach, where hydrochloric acid steps in. Then other enzymes step in at different stages throughout the rest of the process and on down to the end.

Acidic foods and drinks begin neutralizing the enzymes in your saliva right off the bat, interfering with the very first stages of digestion. This is a prime reason to consciously add enzyme laden foods and/or supplements to your diet, especially if you have a chronic illness where your enzymes are notoriously low to begin with.

There are eight types of digestive enzymes, each breaking down specific kinds of foods:

1. Protease: digests protein and helps inflammation

2. Amylase: digests carbohydrates and works as a natural antihistamine

3. Lipase: digests fats and can remove fatty deposits in arteries

4. Cellulase: breaks down fiber

5. Maltase: converts complex sugars from grains and

malt into useable glucose

6. Lactase: digests milk sugar (lactose) in dairy products

7. Phytase: helps overall digestion, and is a key enzyme for bone health

8. Sucrase: digests the sugars found in most foods

All of these (and all the other enzymes) are equally important, of course, but the three heavy hitters who work the hardest are the protease, amylase, and lipase enzymes which work on the protein, carbohydrates, and fats respectively.

Protease. Because protein is a most difficult substance to metabolize, the proteolytic enzymes (proteases) are particularly important. They help to completely digest protein particles that could otherwise create major havoc in a number of ways, most notoriously by punching a hole through the intestinal wall and getting into the bloodstream—a condition called *leaky gut syndrome.* The gluten protein molecule, found in wheat, rye and barley, is a notorious instigator of this condition.[7] But it's clearly not the only one. According to Sayer Ji, author, lecturer, researcher, and founder of GreenMedInfo.com, there are as many as twenty-three thousand other proteins such as gliadins, glutelins, e.g. that can and do cause just as much damage. [8]

The vast majority of metabolic enzymes in the body are, in fact, protease enzymes. Having sufficient proteases is known to help reduce inflammation, and actually clean up waste protein debris in the circulatory system (blood vessels and veins), thereby boosting the immune system and actually helping sinusitis, asthma, allergies, and a number of autoimmune conditions. [9] For more information on the importance of proteolytic enzymes for treating these conditions read Jon Barron's *Lessons from Miracle Doctors* (Basic Health Productions, 2008). Dr. Nicholas Gonzales has followed up with utilizing metabolic enzymatic cancer therapy for healing numerous types of cancer, including pancreatic cancer. [10]

Amylase is the starch-digesting enzyme that helps digest all carbohydrates. It is produced in the pancreas like most of the others, and *also* in the salivary glands. The mouth is where digestion begins, and with carbs being so plentiful in our diet, it is a good thing that amylase is produced here too. A *sufficient amount* of amylase helps reduce inflammation common in osteoarthritis, rheumatoid arthritis, lupus and other autoimmune conditions, and it is found to boost immunomodulatory activity (boost the immune system). Insufficient digestion of carbohydrates has been linked, not only to blood sugar imbalances, but also to allergies and asthma, leading many to consider sufficient amounts of amylase (to allow complete digestion of carbohydrates) a natural antihistamine! [11]

Lipase helps boost the immune system and helps convert good fats to fuel. If you are eating an abundance of unhealthy fried and fatty foods, your limited store of lipase is working overtime, under duress and inefficiently. Consequently, most of these bad fats don't get broken down and end up creating mayhem in the form of fatty deposits in blood vessels, veins, organs and muscles... like the heart muscle! This activity also lowers your store of lipase for working with the good fats that you *do* eat, making these fats ineffectual due to malabsorption because of insufficient lipase. So your small amount of existing lipase is still spinning its wheels trying desperately to digest the hydrogenates and trans fats, while the good fats don't even get a chance.

Good fats are necessary to enable fat-soluble vitamins like A, D, E, and K to become absorbed, but most importantly of all to support the cell walls of *every cell in the body*, making the cells firm, yet malleable and permeable for full functioning. With three different types of lipase, produced in the pancreas, the stomach and the salivary glands, this would indicate the importance of having sufficient quantities. A short supply of lipase can instigate a number of diseases and conditions... obesity, irritable bowel syndrome, bloating, heartburn, indigestion, and celiac disease being only a few. [12]

The remaining digestive enzymes are equally important for breaking down fiber, milk sugars, and other sugars and aiding in general digestion, while also helping in metabolic activity. According to "Smokey" Santillo, ND, "We are maintained not by the food we eat, but by the food we actually digest. Food must be broken down by enzymes into simpler building blocks, or it is useless." [12a]

Metabolic Enzymes

Metabolic enzymes are responsible for the structuring, repair and remodeling of every cell and tissue. As stated earlier, one enzyme works with phosphorous to build bone; another helps coagulate blood when you get a cut; another helps eliminate carbon dioxide from your lungs when you breathe; others help in the construction of new muscle or nerve or skin tissues; others help the liver, kidney, lung and skin in removing waste from the body and on and on. Virtually every single function of *all* of our systems is enabled by enzymes, metabolic enzymes to be specific.

Matt Monarch's article, "Extend Your Life with Enzymes," tells us, "Enzymes taken on an empty stomach serve an incredibly different function than digestion. These enzymes are immediately directed to the metabolic processes of our bodies." Test results prove that enzymes taken on an empty stomach do indeed assist the metabolic functions of our body, including the miraculous repair of any damage sustained by the body. [13]

In other words, depending upon when you take enzyme supplements, you are either aiding your body's digestion, *or* aiding its metabolic processes. So, a snack of fruit or other enzyme-rich food eaten between meals, for example, adds to your metabolic enzyme function. [14] Eating it with a meal will cause the enzymes in that food to be utilized for digestion, thereby saving your own pancreas-created enzymes for later.

Of course the real thing, raw whole foods, is always best, but supplements also add to your stores and help your body increase its own store of enzymes. Supplements can make a great back-up system. [15]

Food Enzymes

Most of us eat dead food, i.e. processed, sugary, fried, and fast foods. These foods destroy enzymes. Overuse of antibiotics and prescription meds do too for that matter. These things not only destroy enzymes, they interfere with your body's efforts to make its own enzymes.

The good news is you can get all the enzymes you need from foods, raw foods specifically, and if necessary from supplements. When you eat sufficient raw foods with enzymes or take enzyme supplements, this allows your body to store its own self-made enzymes for metabolic use, instead of converting them to being used in the digestive process. It's like saving money in the bank for when you really need it. It helps to prevent the exhaustion of your enzyme potential, which could lead to pancreatic breakdown and ultimately to diseases and disorders that can overrun your body before anyone knows what's happening! [16]

Enzymes are the "life force" in raw foods – that God-given spark in the raw food that gives *us* life. Raw food is living food, rich in enzymes and good bacteria (probiotics).

It's interesting to note that foods and liquids at 117 degrees can be touched and handled without a second thought, while foods at 118 degrees and over are painful and can burn you when touched. This is a guide to maintaining enzymes within your food. Below 117 degrees, your raw food is still a life-giving entity. If it's too hot to handle, it's not worth handling, and you'll definitely need to get your enzymes from supplements. Over 118 degrees, the enzymes within are "deactivated" and can no longer serve their purpose. [17]

Raw nuts and seeds contain the enzyme lipase for digesting fats. Nearly all raw fruits and vegetables contain amylase which breaks down carbohydrates. *Sprouted grains, seeds, and beans are practically "pre-digested" with all the activated enzymes in these germinated foods (mostly, proteases). [18]

Bromelain and papain, found in pineapple and papaya respectively, are well known for digesting proteins, but they are also famous for their excellent anti-inflammatory and pain-relieving qualities, too. [19]

Buying Enzyme Supplements

A number of enzyme supplements are sold individually, but to get the most for your dollar, it may be wise to purchase supplemental enzymes in combination. Many well-known, reputable companies provide supplements with a grouping of digestive and metabolic enzymes. Some of these companies are Enzymedica, Garden of Life, Jarrow Formulas, Maximum Living, Metagenics, Natrol, Nature's Bounty, Nature's Sunshine, Now Foods, Standard Process, The Vitamin Shoppe, and others. You can be sure that these enzyme supplements are from actual plant or animal (natural) sources because scientists haven't yet found a way to reproduce them synthetically! Enzymes ARE the life force of the plant or animal, remember.

Note: Please do not take enzymes or enzyme supplements (or *any* supplements, for that matter) with acidic soft drinks, coffee, or alcohol. Orange juice and grapefruit juice are not wise either, due to their acidic nature - the enzymes would be neutralized in the mouth or esophagus before arriving at their destination. Other juices that turn out to be mostly sugar water are not recommended either. Water, is the fluid of choice; or if necessary, herbal tea or almond, rice or coconut milks.

TIP A full glass of clean, clear water (lukewarm water works best) with the juice of a freshly squeezed organic lemon is one of the very best healthy habits you can start today. Lemon

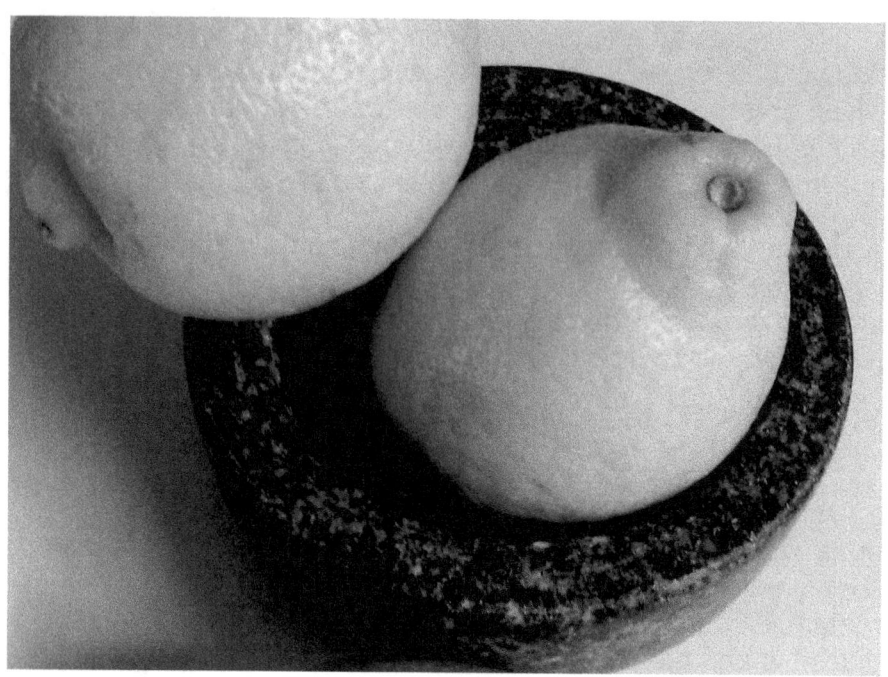

water oxygenates red blood cells, alkalinizes, and helps balance your body's pH, *and* it helps maximize liver enzymes!

Dr. David Jockers tells us, "Lemon is known to stimulate the liver's natural enzymes. This assists the liver in the process of dumping toxins like uric acid and in liquefying congested bile ducts." [20]

Lemon water aids in hydration and adds electrolytes (magnesium, calcium, and potassium) and antioxidants, including vitamin C. It can help dissolve calcium deposits, including kidney and pancreatic stones. It helps reduce phlegm in the body. Drinking lemon water is an excellent way to treat your body well.[21] And it's a great little detox to use first thing every morning, while jump-starting the liver enzymes!

Note: Lime and other citrus fruits are similar in action, but lemon is the most potent.

```
                    Raw enzyme-rich foods


   Pineapple      sprouted grains*           raw honey
   Papaya         sprouted seeds*            raw butter
   Banana         sprouted beans*            raw milk
   Mango          dehydrated fruits and veggies  fermented foods
   Watermelon     garlic                     yogurt
   Cantaloupe     broccoli                   sour cream
   Apple          avocado                    coconut water
   Cabbage        Brussels sprouts           alfalfa
```

Info Box 2

Probiotics

Probiotics are the *good* bacteria that help balance out the bad bacteria. Let's face it, bacteria happens; there's no way to avoid it, especially in warm dark places like the intestine. Ideally, the "good" bacteria should outnumber the "bad" in order to help prevent inflammation, headaches, eczema, psoriasis, respiratory or sinus infections, yeast infections (which can lead to chronic fatigue), vaginitis, bloating, stomach issues, and illnesses like leaky gut syndrome, ulcerative colitis, candidiasis, Crohn's Disease, and more. And you thought probiotics were just used to ease digestion and diarrhea! [22]

Yet, the most important reason we need to add probiotics to our diet is because studies have shown that 80% of our immune system lies in the gut, which is why all these conditions benefit from a healthy gut. The gut has been called "our second brain." We *must* take care to treat it right! It is essential to have good gut flora working *for* us on a daily basis. The bad bacteria always seem to make their way in there, so we must add the good stuff to be sure it all works in our favor! [23]

Case Adams, PhD, ND, alternative medical practitioner at the Watsonville Wellness and Rehabilitation Center in Santa Cruz County, California, and author of *Probiotics: Protection Against Infection* (Logical Books, 2009) writes that researchers at UCLA's Geffen School of Medicine have determined that consuming milk fermented with probiotics changes the brain activity of women— "their task-related responses increased, and their activity within the sensory cortex regions changed… Their midbrain connectivity increased, which the researchers concluded probably explained their task-related response increases." [24] In fact, Adams tells us that there are more than 100 known benefits for taking probiotics. [25] He cites numerous studies showing many of these benefits for many conditions. A short list can be found at Neutraceuticals World.com. [26]

The word "probiotics" generally brings to mind those little cups of yogurt one sees advertised on TV. While helpful in their own way, they do contain food dyes, artificial flavors and preservatives, and of course, sugar—sometimes *lots* of sugar—which makes you want *more* sugar. So when you finish your little cup of yogurt, you often end up scraping the bottom for every last little tiny bit you can squeeze out of it. (FYI, sugar feeds yeast infections and increases inflammation. So if you are eating yogurt to help either of these conditions, any sugar in your yogurt is actually feeding the problem!) And of course aspartame is not a recommended additive for anyone. Much better for you, *and* more effective, is the plain, unsweetened type of yogurt, especially Greek Yogurt. [27]

Unsweetened yogurt has more protein, potassium, calcium, zinc, and vitamins B-6 and B-12 than sweetened yogurt. [28] And it's thicker and creamier. What kind of plain unsweetened yogurt brands are out there? Look for unsweetened Fage®, Mountain High®, Stoneyfield®, Chobani®, Chobani Greek Yogurt®, Organic Oikos®, Trader Joe's® Plain, Wallaby

Organic Plain Regular Yogurt®, and Wallaby plain Greek Yogurt®. [29]

Always read the label. Be sure it contains "live cultures." See if sugar *or* aspartame or any other sweeteners are listed. For our purposes, zero is best, or aim at yogurts with the smallest amount of sugar possible (see the recommended brands above). Yogurt can be sweetened at home with fresh bananas, strawberries, blueberries, dried tart cherries, pineapple, cranberries, raisins, currants, raw honey, real maple syrup, cinnamon, molasses, or even dehydrated cane sugar (Sucanant) or Stevia.

I recommend buying the low fat yogurt or even the full fat yogurt, which uses whole milk and cultures. Because the full fat yogurt has a richer, creamier, more satisfying, taste, you stay fuller longer. This is healthy fat; good for you; full of vitamins A and D. It can be hard to find, but it's worth it for the creaminess, flavor, and satiety! If the fat factor goes against your grain

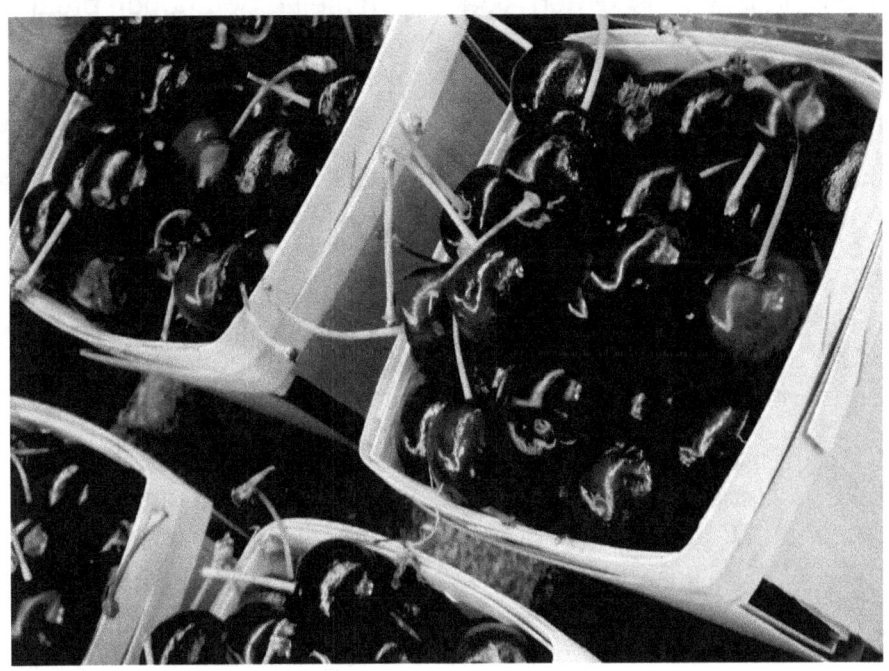

through past conditioning, then go with the *low*-fat. The "no fat" edition inevitably adds a sugar (or two or three, with a variety of names) or aspartame and "other flavors" along with tapioca or cornstarch, and all sorts of things to give it a semblance of real flavor in place of the missing good, whole milk fat. Read the label.[30]

For those folks who are lactose intolerant, or those who have a protein allergy to milk and certain dairy product, you don't necessarily need to avoid yogurt. Except for those with severe allergies, many can still eat yogurt. During the culturing process the live active cultures actually create the enzyme lactase. And according to Dr. William Sears and wife, Martha Sears, RN at Askdrsears.com, "Bacterial enzymes created by the culturing process, partially digest the milk protein casein, making it easier to absorb and less allergenic." [30a, 31]

Yogurt is not the only way to get probiotics, of course. There are supplements, and fermented foods like pickles, Sauerkraut, miso, Kimchi, Kefir, buttermilk, Kombucha tea, as well as algae like Spirulina, Blue-Green Algae or Chlorella. Sourdough bread has probiotics, but be aware that when toasted or heated, a lot of the good probiotics are destroyed. [32]   There are even probiotics mixed into chocolate. [33]

Deirdre Rawlings, PhD, ND, MH, CNC has written an excellent and very helpful book, with recipes, titled, *Fermented Foods for Health: Use the Power of Probiotic Foods to Improve Your Digestion, Strengthen Your Immunity, and Prevent Illness* (Fair Winds Press 2013). The title says it all! Another article by Mark Sisson, "The Definitive Guide to Fermented Foods," can be found on his excellent website, Marksdailyapple.com.[34]

Although there are more than 500 strains of probiotics, and billions of individual bacteria within those strains adding up to more than 3 trillion organisms, it's amazing to note that each probiotic strain promotes optimal health in a distinctly different manner. Lactobacillus and Bifidobacterium are the two most common strains, the former residing mostly in the intestine and the latter mostly everywhere from head to toe, like the other 498 strains. [35, 36]

If you have been using antibiotics, you are especially in need of replenishing your stores of good bacteria. Most Health Care Practitioners (HCP) prefer you wait until you have completed your antibiotic regimen; then, begin adding a good unsweetened probiotic daily and regularly. Other HCP's will suggest taking the probiotic immediately an hour or two after taking the antibiotic. Some probiotics in the gut are pretty hardy and can withstand some assault from the antibiotics for a short time, but replenishing them is still necessary for overall good gut health.

Zach C. Miller's article, "Health is Directly Linked to the Gut: Eleven Things that Destroy the Beneficial Probiotic Bacteria Living Inside Us," found at the *Natural News* website, puts antibiotics right at the top of this list of eleven. Also listed in his article as "things to avoid" that destroy our friendly probiotics are: Chlorine, Fluoride, coffee, carbonated beverages, radiation, pesticides and … yes, STRESS! [37]

Buying probiotic Supplements

For those who wish to utilize the convenience of supplements, whether you cannot eat fermented foods or yogurts or if you're traveling and need a portable probiotic, there are a few things to look for when buying these supplements.

It is helpful to check with a third-party testing facility like ConsumerLab.com where they test the viability, quality and quantity of many supplements every year, randomly and regularly. [38] In the case of probiotics, they also test the actual active live cultures after being activated to verify that the listed number of billions remains.

Stick to well-known brand names. Popular accepted brand names that have been listed at Consumer Lab in the past have been Align® Digestive Care, Culturelle® Natural Health & Wellness, Dr. Ohhira's Probiotic®, Garden of Life® RAW Probiotic for Women, GNC® Ultra 75 Probiotic Complex, Jarro-Dophilus EPS®, Metagenics® Ultra Flora Plus, Nature's Bounty® Probiotics, Nature's Way® Primadophilus Optima, Puritan's Pride®, Vitamin Shoppe® Ultimate 10 Probiotic, Vitamin World®, and Walgreens Finest® Digestive Probiotics.

The specific strains you choose can make a difference. They are all work-specific – each strain working on a specific task, all helping to balance our gut. [39]

- Lactobacillus (acidophilus, casei, plantarum, etc.)

- Bifidobacterium (bifidum, infantis, lactis, etc.)

- Streptococcus (thermopiles)

- Lactococcus (lactis)

- Enterococcus (faecium) and more.

You can choose a single strain in your purchase, such as Lactobacillus acidophilus, or you may choose two or three strains, or even a whole menagerie! Choosing several in one capsule seems to be a bit more effective for overall health as they cover more territory, each in their own way. The Garden Of Life® RAW Probiotic for Women, for example lists 25 or more types of several strains, and Nature's Way® Primadophilus

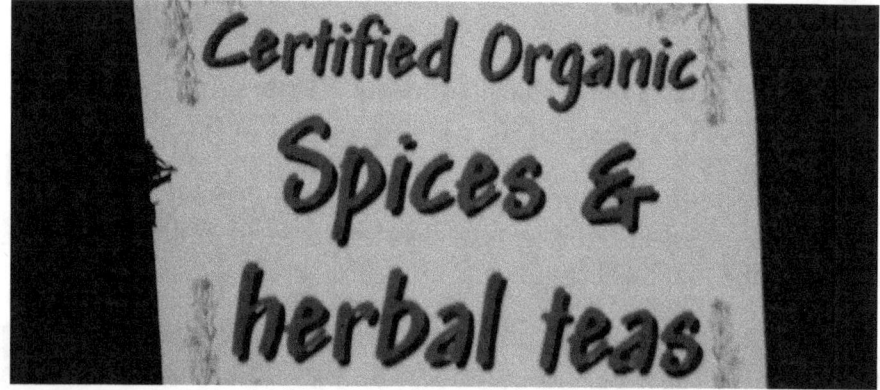

Optima has 13 types of a few strains.

When reading the label, always check "other ingredients" beneath the actual box of listed ingredients. Be certain there are no allergic items listed such as soy, egg, wheat, nuts, etc. that you may have a reaction to.

Check bacterial counts. Don't buy any less than 1 billion CFUs (Colony Forming Units). A maintenance dose for *healthy* folks would be 3-5 billion CFUs per day. Therapeutic doses can exceed 1 trillion per day. [40]

Look for a probiotic with an *enteric-coating*. This protects the probiotic from being dissolved by the stomach's hydrochloric acid before it gets to your intestine where it does the work.

Some probiotics are found in the refrigerator section of your local health food store and must continue to be refrigerated at home—these are live active cultures. The probiotics found on the shelf are in a dormant, inactive state after being freeze-dried and will be "activated" by the heat of your body once ingested. These should not be exposed to heat before you take them. They should be kept in a cool, dry, and dark place.

Follow the directions on the label unless your Health Care Physician tells you otherwise. Some recommend one per day, others two per day; some recommend taking with meals, others between meals—follow the recommendations listed. Also, don't forget to check the expiration date.

TIP ONE Plain unsweetened yogurt doesn't have to be a stand-alone food. Yogurt is great in a smoothie, mixed into oatmeal, or as a substitute for milk in dry cereal or granola. Substitute for sour cream and on top of a baked potato or a taco. Substitute for mayonnaise in your tuna or chicken salad. Spread it on top of a bagel or muffin. Mix it with raw honey and spread on a muffin or eat it as is. Put it in the freezer and ½ hour later eat it like ice cream! Make delicious dips by adding avocado; or onion, sea salt, pepper, and a bit of red-wine vinegar; or olive oil, sea salt and oregano.

TIP TWO What's the difference between Greek yogurt and regular yogurt? Which is better? Both have roughly the same amount of calories. Greek yogurt has more protein, usually double that of regular yogurt. It's more filling for a longer period. Greek yogurt has fewer carbohydrates. Also, because of the way it's made, there is even less of the milk sugar, lactose. [41]

Prebiotics

Prebiotics (aka the fiber part of foods) are the nourishment that stimulates the growth and activity of *probiotics*—they are food for the good bacteria. Bad bacteria ignore them. Prebiotics are essentially non-digestible foods, or fiber. They can go right on through to the intestine and feed the good bacteria, mainly Lactobacillus and Bifidobacterium in order to get the job done! [42]

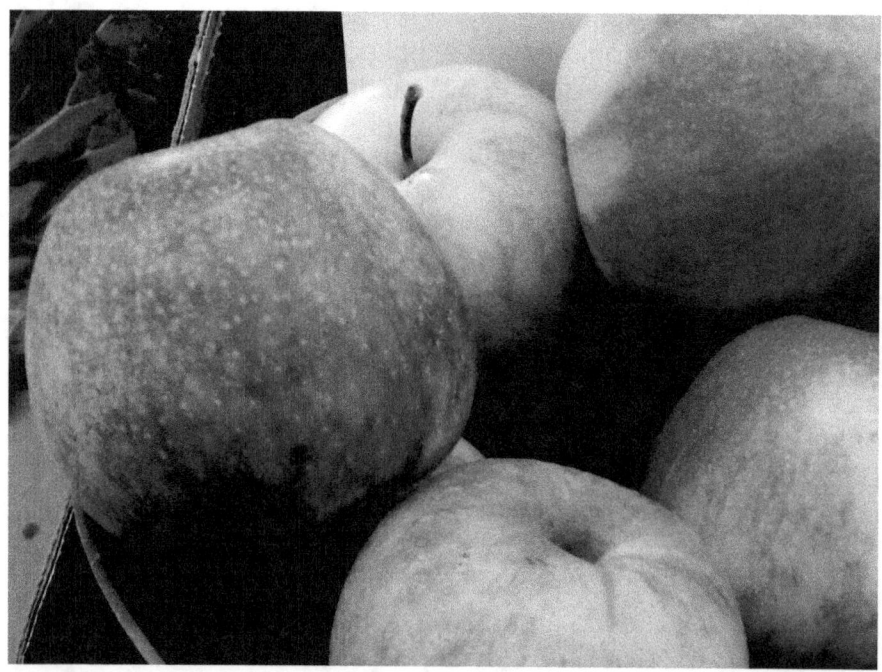

Pati Chandler

Prebiotics are found in foods like apples, bananas and berries, garlic and onion, Jerusalem artichokes and asparagus, leafy greens and legumes, oats and barley, kidney beans, chicory root and dandelion root, real maple syrup and raw honey, raw apple cider and much more. Prebiotics are often added to probiotic supplements to enhance absorption and activity. [43]

They even have stand-alone health benefits! According to a report done by 20 international experts written in the August 2010 edition of the *British Journal of Nutrition*, the following health benefits of prebiotics have been established in both animal and human studies:

- Increased calcium absorption

- Enhanced immune function

- Stronger and healthier balance in the gut

- Normalized bowel function

- Reduction of leaky gut and toxins

- Appetite suppression

- Reduced risk of intestinal infection

More studies are being done as we speak, resulting from the evidence in these tests.

Prebiotics have proven to help cholesterol and triglyceride levels, and according to one study they can reduce atherosclerosis (hardening of the arteries) by 30%, thereby significantly helping heart health. [44]

Because we now know that 80% of our immune system lies in the gut, it is to our great benefit to maintain a healthy well-balanced beneficial bacterial gut. Wiping out pathogens and bad bacteria in the gut can help a whole host of issues, including Crohn's Disease and other inflammatory bowel issues, as well as many other conditions. It may even prove useful for treating cancer, osteoporosis, and diabetes! [45]

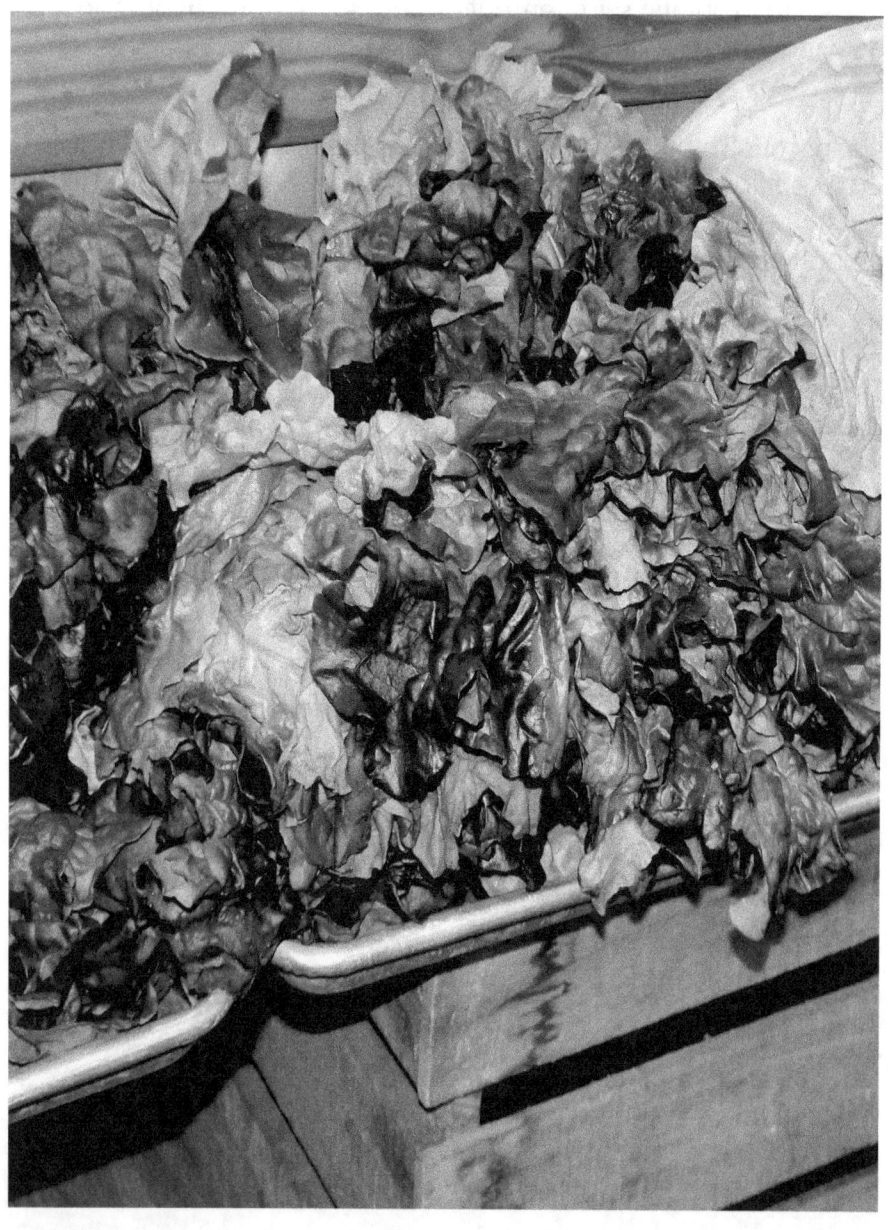

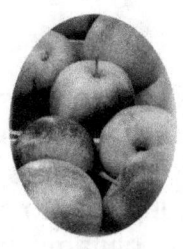

Chapter 3

Proteins

Meats are the first thing that comes to mind when we think of protein—beef generally, then maybe turkey or chicken (these are our best sources for B-12 too), then we might think of fish, then eggs and dairy. It's true; all of these are our very best sources of protein. However, proteins are also found in nuts, beans, seeds, grains, and more.

Proteins are not stored in our body like fats or carbohydrates, and so it is essential to eat proteins for our health and well-being, every single day – some protein at each meal would be ideal. Why is protein essential? Because all of the following are made up of proteins: enzymes, antibodies, hormones, hemoglobin (blood), neurotransmitters, ligaments, muscle (including the heart muscle), bones, hair, nails, and skin. In fact, proteins are the basic component of *every cell* in every living body! [1] Yes, we need protein to survive.

What kinds of proteins do we need?

Proteins are composed of 20 different kinds of amino acids, divided into two forms – essential amino acids, which we need to add in our diet, and non-essential amino acids that our body can produce as long as we have a sufficient supply of the components necessary to do so.

Many of us with a chronic illness find ourselves fairly low in one or more of these components, *or* low in the enzymes required to carry out the process of producing them; sometimes, even both! Some examples of these non-essential aminos which our body is supposed to supply would be: cysteine, tyrosine, glutamine, glutamic acid, aspartic acid, and others. If our body is not supplying the proper amounts of these aminos, then this would affect the quantity, quality, and function of our enzymes in addition to hormones, neurotransmitters, and our every cell. Obviously this affects our metabolic and physiological processes. Some may even find it necessary *to add them to their diet.* [2, 3]

Foods containing proteins are classified as "complete" or "incomplete" protein sources. Meat, fish, fowl, and dairy sources are complete proteins containing a balance of all 20 amino acids. Incomplete proteins are plant and vegetable proteins which are lacking one or more of the necessary 20 amino acids. So to get the proper balance via plant sources alone, one must plan which protein foods to combine throughout the day in order to acquire the necessary 20 aminos.

Excellent sources of complete proteins (animal): Wild turkey*, venison*, free-range chicken*, grass-fed beef*, buffalo*, lamb, pork loin, pork chops, free-range (or cage-free) eggs*, cheese, cottage cheese, yogurt, tuna, salmon, halibut, cod, sardines, mackerel, shrimp, scallops.

*These are generally low-fat meats and eggs. The fats that *are* found in these meats and eggs are the healthy, anti-inflammatory Omega 3 EPA-DHA fatty acids, and are every bit as healthy and good for you as a slab of salmon. These critters have never been fed man-processed grain.

Regular grocery-store-bought turkey, chicken, and beef,

and such should be as low-fat as you possibly can find. Avoiding meats with excess saturated fats is paramount. The processed grains that are fed to these latter animals make their fat saturated and full of Omega 6 *pro*-inflammatory fatty acids, devoid of any healthy Omega 3 fats. This also makes them more acidic.

Another good complete protein source would be Whey Protein Drinks, available in powder form. Organic is best. Of course, check the label to see if there is any sensitivity or allergic items, like egg, soy, nuts, wheat/gluten, etc. Whey Protein Drinks make an excellent smoothie in the morning mixed with almond or coconut milk and berries or bananas. You can use your imagination here – get creative! They often come in chocolate too!

Note: I don't recommend soy protein drinks, due to their potential effect on the thyroid, and the fact that 90% of this soy is genetically modified.

Excellent sources of incomplete proteins (plant): Beans (kidney, black, pinto, garbanzo), lentils, legumes (peanuts, e.g.), nuts and nut butters (almond, cashew, walnut), seeds

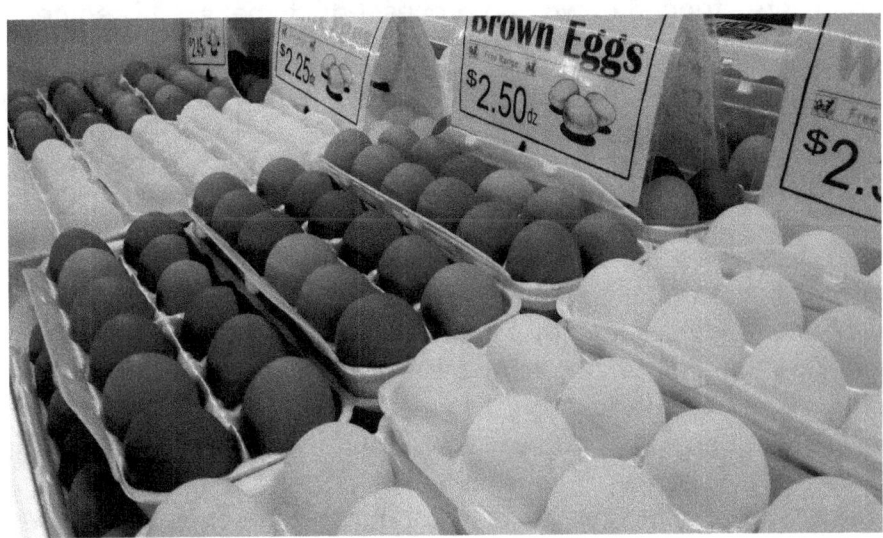

(sesame and sunflower), wild rice, chlorella, spirulina, seaweed, chia seeds, spinach, kale, quinoa*, whole grains** (such as amaranth, buckwheat, oats, spelt and millet), sprouted grains and seeds***. [4]

Wheat protein/gluten is a whole other matter. See "Gluten" in Part 1. Also you may be interested in reading Jonathan Benson's article, "Wheat Contains Over 23,000 Potentially Harmful Proteins," at Natural News.com, complete with references. [5]

*Quinoa is a whole grain that is the exception to the rule – it is a plant that is a complete protein containing all 20 amino acids. A half cup of quinoa has 9 full grams of complete protein; it's loaded with fiber, minerals, and antioxidants; and it's gluten-free! Check George Mateljan's website The World's Healthiest Foods, for loads of details and recipes! [6,7]

**Whole grains include the whole seed, or kernel, of the plant—the bran, germ, and endosperm. The bran contains antioxidants, B-vitamins, and fiber. The germ contains more B-vitamins, some protein, minerals, and healthy Omega 3 fatty acids. The endosperm contains starchy carbohydrates, a little protein, and a small amount of vitamins and minerals. When grains are stripped down and processed, all that's left is some of the endosperm, and not a whole lot of its beneficial protein and minerals, leaving none of the good fatty acids. In fact, seventeen vitamins and minerals are gone, along with 25% of its protein. [8]

***Sprouted grains are whole grains that have been sprouted. These sprouts are literally "new life" from the grain, and they contain all the life nutrients, enzymes, proteins, vitamins, minerals, etc. that they will need to grow into a whole plant. Holistic nutritionist, Karen Foster tells us that sprouted foods are "…a living food that metabolically works with the human body effortlessly." See her excellent article at PreventDisease.com, "12 Reasons to Eat Sprouts, a Living Food with Amazing Health Benefits" where she explains their benefits and shows how to sprout your own foods for really fresh food health benefits! [9]

Sprouted grain breads are actually called "flourless bread." The sprouts of wheat, spelt, millet, rye, barley, rice, quinoa, peas, lentils, beans, seeds (sunflower, sesame, etc.) are ground or mashed into a kind of puree, and then pressed into their final shape – muffin, bread, buns, pasta, tortilla, cereal, and such. These are the freshest kind of foods and are necessarily found in the freezer section of your health food store. You can also buy sprouted grain "flour" to make your own dishes. [10]

Sprouting releases enzyme inhibitors, so ultimately there can be up to 100 times more enzymes in your sprouted foods than in uncooked fruits and veggies. Sprouting also helps make all the vitamins, minerals, amino acids, and essential fatty acids in your foods highly absorbable. [11]

I am sensitive to gluten in regular breads, but I have no trouble at all with the *Food For Life®* brand "7-Sprouted Grain English Muffins" or their "Cinnamon Raisin Muffins" five mornings a week for breakfast! [12]

Note: For those with more severe reactions like complete intolerance to wheat/gluten or those with celiac, these products may not be right for you. Please talk to your health care provider. Food For Life® Company also makes gluten-free breads.

Original soy (not GMO) is also an exception to the rule, and is considered a complete protein. But fermented soy is the only way it should be eaten, and I do highly recommend it. Natto, miso, and tempeh are excellent forms of soy, aka fermented foods. They are top-notch probiotic foods and full of all the amino acids required to be a called a complete protein. However, soy found in packaged foods (even in health bars and Tofu, which is not fermented) is: 1) 90% or more genetically modified (GMO) and 2) a goitrogen, well-known to interfere with thyroid function. Therefore, I don't recommend eating soy found in packaged products or soy nuts. [13]

How much protein do we need?

People in developed countries rarely need to worry about *not* getting enough protein. However, there is a bone of contention as to how much protein is optimal for everyone. It is really not possible to say that this or that amount of protein is right for everyone. Ideally, we should each find what works best for our individual body, considering age, weight, activity level, medical condition, and special circumstances. Most nutritionists recommend eating some protein with each meal (some healthy fats and complex carbs with each meal too, by the way) for a well-rounded, fulfilling meal that lasts until the next meal. [14] Protein helps to make you feel fuller longer because it takes longer for your stomach and intestines to fully process and digest protein than fats and carbs.

According to the CDC (Centers for Disease Control) 10-35% of a 2,000 calorie daily diet should consist of protein. The 35% would be recommended for a healthy young athlete and 10% for those who are more sedentary. This recommendation includes women and men ages 19-70+, no matter the shape, size, or health condition of the individual. This is about 46 grams per day for women and 56 grams per day for men. [15] I find this recommendation to be inadequate. The age range alone is so broad as to be meaningless.

Miriam Nelson's article, "Find Out How Consuming Too Much Protein Can Harm Your Body," a WebMD Feature on MedicneNet.com, explains recommendations from the Food and Nutrition Board in body weight and grams. "Ideally, you should consume 0.36 grams of protein for every pound of body weight, according to recommended daily allowances (RDA) set by the Food and Nutrition Board. So if you weigh 170 pounds, you need about 61 grams of protein each day." [16] It's not easy to gauge how many grams of what you are eating.

```
+------------------------------------------------------------------+
|               A sampling of protein amounts.                     |
|             Read labels for more information                     |
|                                                                  |
|                                                                  |
|  1 cup of milk                   = 8 grams of protein            |
|  1medium egg                     = 6.7 grams                     |
|  1 sprouted grain muffin         = 8 grams                       |
|  1 small (3 oz.) piece of meat   = 21 grams                      |
|  1 average (8 oz.) piece of meat = 50 grams                      |
|  1 (5 oz.) can of tuna           = 13 grams                      |
|  ½ cup of cooked dry beans       = 8 grams                       |
|  2 tbs. Peanut butter            = 7 grams                       |
|  1 (8 oz.) Greek yogurt          = 11 grams                      |
|  1 (6 oz.) Yoplait               = 5 grams                       |
|  1 (5.8 oz.) low fat ice cream   = 4 grams                       |
|                                                                  |
+------------------------------------------------------------------+
```

Info Box 3

The National Institute of Health's MedlinePlus' website recommendation of "two to three servings of protein-rich foods per day" is much more realistic, and I lean more toward the three per day—it's easier to calculate than grams per body weight. [17]

The idea is to find what works best for you. I tend to do best with the nutritionists' recommendations and snack on a yogurt or a couple of tsp. of crunchy peanut butter or a handful of nuts in between meals if my activity level warrants it.

If you take a look at the list above, you could see where the CDC's recommended 46 grams of protein per day could easily be acquired by eating a number of proteins throughout the day. You could eat at least one protein with each meal by mixing and matching a number of the items above. The important thing to remember would be to keep the portion size realistic. Your choice of lean meat, for example should be 2 or 3 ounces, or about the size of a deck of playing cards. [18] Definitely include at least a few pieces of lean meat per week, not only for the protein, but also for the necessary B-12 in your diet. Then add beans, yogurt, eggs, tuna, peanut butter, or other proteins to give an interesting variety to your diet.

If you don't get enough protein in the food you eat, your body will begin to breakdown its own muscle to support its need for amino acids! [19] Eating only 50 -75% of the daily requirement can create a deficiency. [20]   And it's important to be sure that the protein you *do* eat is digestible and absorbable. It's actually possible to eat an abundant amount of protein and yet still "starve" for amino acids! Think "protease enzymes" here, to go with the complete proteins to aid in absorption.

Too much protein is not necessarily beneficial either. Gail Butterfield, PhD, RD, director of Nutrition Studies at the Palo Alto Veterans' Administration Medical Center and nutrition lecturer at Stanford University, tells that "...consuming too much protein—more than 30% of your total daily caloric intake, could actually harm your body." [21]

In a recent study into potential causes of pre-diabetes at the National Institute of Health in Tokyo, it was found that a high intake of protein and low levels of minerals (an acid-

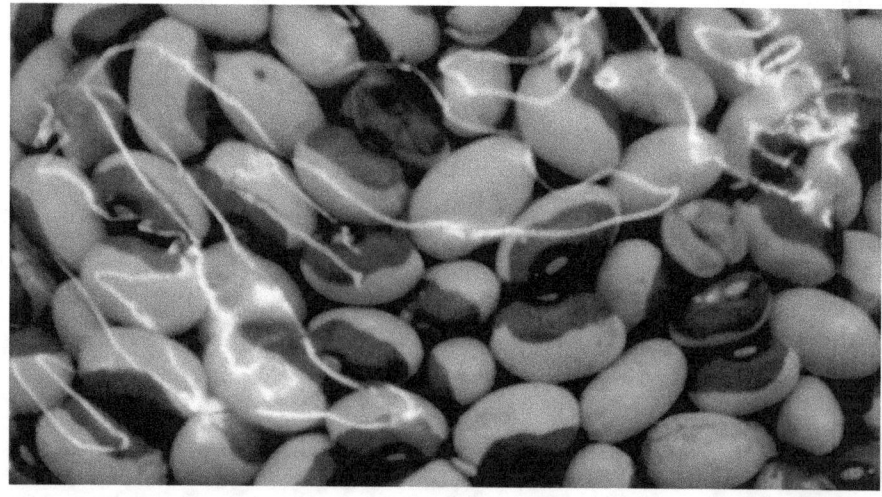

forming diet) resulted in a condition called metabolic acidosis. Acid-forming diets are those with more than 25% of calories from fat and more than 75 grams of total daily protein. All this protein and fat makes a body quite full, resulting in a reduction of fiber, vitamins and minerals found in the alkaline-forming fruits, veggies, nuts, seeds and whole grains. Ultimately, this in turn leads to a body being overfed, undernourished, and in a state of metabolic acidosis. High acidity has been shown to lead to many, if not all, chronic, inflammatory, degenerative, autoimmune conditions. [22]

It's true; packing in protein in a short amount of time has been shown to aid in weight loss. However, doing this indefinitely can cause major consequences. Initially, minor side-effects can include headaches, dizziness, confusion, fatigue, and nausea. Then there's the concern about high cholesterol and gout. Long term excess protein can put a huge amount of stress on the kidneys and create a loss in bone density by forcing the body to pull calcium from bones to help alkalinize the acidic load in your body. [23]

Those who eat excess protein run the risk of cutting back too much on fats, fiber, and carbohydrates. These would be the same complex carbohydrates that contain the necessary enzymes for the digestion of those proteins; the same fiber that allows the bowels to keep things in motion, which can be a challenge with too much protein. There may be a risk of too much animal saturated fats that are *not* good, so it's important to focus on the foods with good fats that accompany the protein – i.e. salmon, free-range beef, buffalo, lean meats, and vegetable fats, like coconut oil and avocados.

Balance, *in the appropriate portions*, is the thing. Richard Collins, MD, FACC (aka The Cooking Cardiologist) recommends a plate that might look like a three section dish of 25%, 25% and 50% of protein, fats, and carbohydrates, respectively. [24]   There would be an overlap, of course, so don't expect to use an actual divided plate. For example, salmon will supply not only your protein but also some of the good fats.

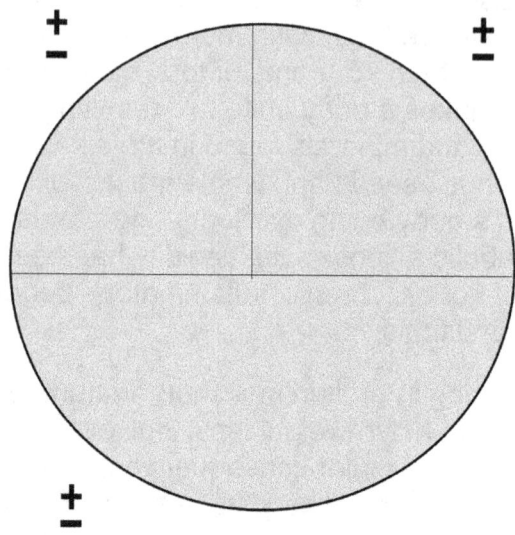

Fig. 2

Also, consider making tuna salad with a tablespoon of coconut oil instead of mayonnaise; that will add even more good fats to the tuna protein. A chicken and avocado salad with olive oil drizzled over it will make a delicious meal. Then the idea is to fill the other half of your plate with complex carbohydrates – veggies, greens, whole grains, lentils or beans, maybe slivered almonds or other nuts. You get the idea.

I would recommend a "Plus or Minus" sign at each section so these percentages would be adjustable and flexible for each person as to height, weight, age, physical and medical condition in addition to the particular meal: breakfast, lunch, or dinner. But try to keep the proteins and fats sections between a solid 20-25%! Saturated fats are included here, by the way, but should consist of only about 7-8% within the 20-25% fats section of the pie.

[TIP] Proteins and fats help balance sugar, aka carbs. This is especially important for diabetics. For all of us, even if you

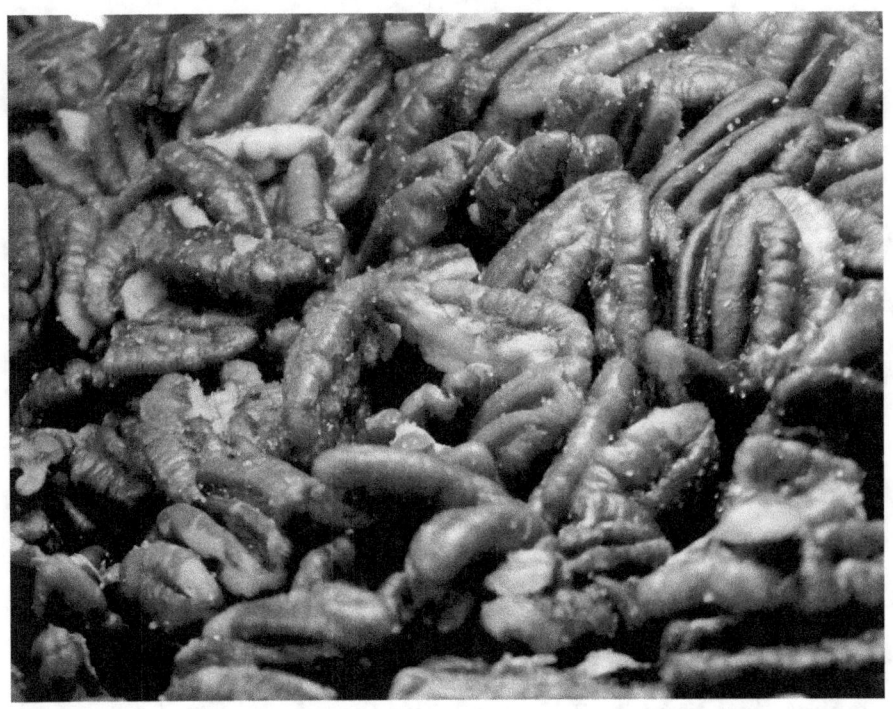

find it difficult to stick to the above percentages, it is extremely important to have at least *some* protein and good fats along with your healthy complex carbs at every meal. They work together in the body. When these foods are eaten individually on a regular basis, they can throw a body out of balance in a hurry – in the form of acidosis, ketosis, diabetes, stomach issues, heart issues, and many more autoimmune conditions. Balance is the key.

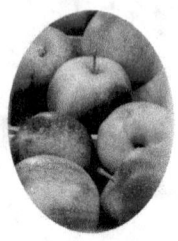

Chapter 4

Fats

Most of this generation has grown up with a severe fat phobia. In the early 1950s when the powers that be made a blanket statement that "Fats are bad for you," we took it to heart, so to speak, and blindly followed their recommendations, deleting fats *of all kinds* from our diet – the bad fats *and* the good fats. The grocery shelves and refrigerator cases became filled to the brim with a huge variety of "low-fat" and "fat-free" foods. I feel this blanket announcement was a huge disservice to the entire population.

We have suffered for this obedience in so many ways – mainly through a myriad of chronic illnesses that could have been avoided or at least greatly diminished. Our bodies need fat every bit as much as they need proteins and carbs, or oxygen and water, for that matter. We just need fats in the appropriate amounts, *and* we need the right kinds of fats. In other words, the most important thing to remember about fats is to choose wisely, but *choose*!

Little has been gained over the decades from low-fat eating because people began eating more and more refined carbs, white rice, potatoes, French fries, snack foods, donuts, breads, muffins, fried & sugary foods, and drinks just to get that "full" feeling that they used to get from a reasonable amount of healthy fats found in whole real foods.

> *The most important thing to remember about fats is to choose wisely, but choose!*

These dismal substitute food items are loaded with hydrogenated and trans-fats, not to mention simple carbs and sugars. Most people don't recognize these hydrogenates and trans-fats because they come in the guise of processed sunflower oil, safflower, canola, soybean, corn oil, and so on. These oils have been processed in order to preserve the packaged food item. Processing, you understand, means that it has been cooked to within an inch of its life, making it now hydrogenated or trans-fat oil, filled with free radicals.

A Harvard research article posted in the September 13, 2013 *Huffington Post*, titled, "Why do we overeat? Harvard researchers address obesity and the toxic food environment" states, "Two-thirds of Americans are now overweight and five percent of American children can now be considered 'severely obese,' which puts their health at grave risk." [1, 2]

Dr. Mercola's updated information is even scarier! "Childhood obesity has more than doubled in young children and tripled in adolescents over the past 30 years; 18 percent of American children between the ages of six and 11 now fall in the obese category." [3]

These statistics are abominable. And here we are, still eating low-fat foods. What's wrong with this picture? This concept is obviously *not* working!

In fact, Sweden is the first country to totally delete its "low-fat dogma." Others to follow soon, I pray! According to *Health Impact News*, Sweden's independent committee comprised of doctors and other health experts determined this "low-fat concept" to be total quackery! "This committee, known as the Swedish Council on Health Technology Assessment, pored through tens of thousands of studies published on the subject through May 31, 2013, to arrive at this conclusion, which corroborates with what many in the natural health community have been saying for years." [4]

The Women's Health Initiative Dietary Modification Trial published a study in the February 8, 2006 *Journal of the American Medical Association*. This was an 8-year study involving 49,000 women that found virtually identical rates of heart attack, stroke, and other forms of cardiovascular disease in women who followed a low-fat diet and those who didn't. In addition to that, they also found that women on the low-fat diet didn't lose – or gain – any more weight than women who followed their usual diets. [5]

In the 1960s, 45% of our diet consisted of [mostly healthy] fats and oils and 13% of adults were obese with 1% suffering type-2 diabetes. Today, 33% of our diet consists of fats and oils, yet 34% of adults are obese and 11% suffer type-2 diabetes! Clearly cutting fats and avoiding things like real butter, eggs, nuts, nut butters, coconut oil, etc. has *not* had the desired effect! We're filling up on hydrogenated and trans fat foods loaded with simple carbs so we can get that "full" feeling!
[6]

Saturated fats, especially, got a bad reputation during this decades-long ban on fats. However, new studies are completely reversing this old, inaccurate, incomplete and selective information.

Ronald M. Kraus, MD, is a lipid specialist (fats are a sub-group of lipids) and the director of atherosclerosis research at the Children's Hospital Oakland Research Institute. He and his colleagues have reviewed over 21 studies involving

350,000 people who were tracked for up to 23 years. Their conclusions were published in the *American Journal of Clinical Nutrition*: "People who consumed the most saturated fat *did not* have a higher risk of heart disease, stroke, or any other form of CVD." He further states, "Saturated fat may have an effect on cardiovascular disease (CVD) risk, but the effect is so small that we just can't detect it. We shouldn't be demonizing saturated fat." [7]

It seems that the main reason the medical profession became "anti-saturated fats" is because of the company they keep. Saturated fats always seem to be found in conjunction with loads of sugars, refined carbs, and trans fats along with a huge over-abundance of fatty red meats. [8]

Serving sizes have practically quadrupled! The current population seems to think that a quarter pound of bacon or sausage, a half-pound hamburger or a 12-ounce steak should be the norm for breakfast, lunch, and dinner every day. These are mega-portions! Be realistic. Think balance! Think: a meat serving the size of the palm of your hand or a deck of cards.

We absolutely need proteins. We absolutely need fats. We absolutely need carbohydrates. But let's get real, here! Paying attention to portion sizes and the 25/25/50% general guideline for balance will give you a good head start on where to begin. (See Fig. 2 for balance guideline.)

Why do we need fats?

Vitamins A, D, E, and K can only be absorbed by using fats – not water. There are in fact, many nutrients in fruits and veggies that need fats for human metabolism.[9] Fats coat the wall of every cell in your body, making the cell wall permeable, malleable, functional containers allowing all the nutrients and oxygen to get inside each cell, and the waste to get *out*. Fats enable nerve transmission in the brain and throughout the body; they are good conductors. They not only help produce hormones, fats also help hormones function efficiently. Fats cleanse and lubricate the body – joints, tendons, organs, skin, hair, nails and more. They add to our satiety and help us feel full after we eat, instead of getting hungry an hour later. Fats protect our organs and insulate our body in all kinds of weather. Plant-based fats like avocados, walnuts, olives, flax seeds, etc. have been shown to offer many health benefits, including helping the fight against breast, prostate, and colon cancers. Fish oil fatty acids have been proven to fight inflammation, depression, joint pain, mental acuity, ADHD, macular degeneration, heart disease, and much more. Coconut oil's plant saturated fats are antibiotic, antiviral, antifungal, anti-parasitic, antimicrobial, anti-inflammatory, antioxidant –it heals inflammatory bowel conditions, the MRSA virus, pneumonia, Candida, and it kills cancer cells! Oh yes, we *definitely* need fats!

How to Avoid the Bad Fats

By now you are fully aware that excess animal-based saturated fats, hydrogenated fats and trans fats (partially-hydrogenates) are downright detrimental to a human body. [10]

It's hard to get away from them *all* however, so the key is to learn how to avoid the greatest bulk of the bad fats and learn how to add the healthy, healing fats.

Reading labels helps to avoid a lot of the bad fats. Bottles, jars, boxes, and frozen packages all list their ingredients. Remember to check out the details here. Peanut butters, salad dressings, ketchup, crackers, cereals, nearly everything on the inner aisles of the grocery store are literally loaded with hydrogenates. Look for words like hydrogenated, of course, and partially hydrogenated (aka trans fats), but also the supposedly innocent oils like sunflower, safflower, canola, soybean, and corn oil. *Before* cooking and processing, these oils may have been healthy, but not anymore. Once they are put into the cracker, cookie, cereal, salad dressing, catsup, etc. Dr. Jekyll turns into Mr. Hyde, and now these oils are morphed into hydrogenated and trans fats!

Shopping wisely is the way to go. After reading these labels, you'll be surprised just how often you are eating these inflammation-making hydrogenates.

There are peanut butters, and other nut butters without hydrogenated oils, right there on those shelves. Mara Natha® almond and peanut butters and Smart Balance® Peanut Butters are two brands that have no hydrogenates. They list pure organic cane sugar and/or molasses for their healthy sweeteners. Natural Jif® and Skippy Natural® have no hydrogenates, and list sugar as their second ingredient. For the purists, there are more at your local health food store, which list "peanuts" as their only ingredient. There are many crackers, cereals, corn chips, popcorn, breads, and salad dressings at your health food store that have no hydrogenates. The key is reading labels.

A new study by the Breast *Cancer Research Treatment* team in September 2013 indicates that adolescent girls who regularly eat vegetable proteins such as peanut butter have a much lower risk of breast cancer! "Girls with a family history of breast cancer had significantly lower risk if they consumed these foods or vegetable fat. In conclusion, consumption of vegetable protein, fat, peanut butter, or nuts by older girls may help reduce their risk of BBD as young women." So why not make it *healthy* peanut butter to give an extra edge? [11]

As for animal saturated fats, some is good, a lot is *not*. It's as simple as that. [12] When buying your meats (whole meats, not processed, like hot dogs, bologna etc.), don't be afraid to choose meats with *some* marbling and visible fats, just don't go overboard. The key is in the serving size. A piece of beef or chicken or pork the size of the palm of your hand is ideal. And if you have veggies and leafy greens with it, they will help metabolize the fats.

Dietary fat is necessary for the absorption of nutrients

from fruits and vegetables. In a fascinating study, people who consumed salads with fat-free salad dressing absorbed far less of the helpful nutrients and vitamins from spinach, lettuce, tomatoes, and carrots than those who consumed their salads with a salad dressing containing fat! [13] Do you see how they all work together? All three are needed at each meal: proteins, fats and carbohydrates. They each help the other to get absorbed!

Butter – even lard? Sure! Again, it's a matter of serving size. Using 2 tablespoons per meal is completely acceptable... encouraged!

The Good Fats

Adding good fats to your diet is healing. But you have to actually do it. Healthy fats should be eaten with every meal. Make a point of adding 3 from this list every day.

- A half an avocado, 8-10 olives

- Nuts— ¼ cups of nuts – walnuts, cashews, almonds, pecans, hazelnuts, pistachios

- Nut Butters – 2 tbs. peanut, almond, cashew, hazelnut, sunflower, tahini

- Seeds –3 tbs. flaxseed, Chia seeds, sunflower seeds, pumpkin seeds, hemp seeds

- Butter, tallow (from beef), lard (from pork) - 2 tbs.

- Whole Cheeses, raw milk cheeses –organic, from grass-fed beef, goat, sheep—Cheddar, Colby, Swiss, Parmesan (hard), Edam, Gouda, Feta (check for high salt)

- Fish – 3-5 oz. Salmon, Tuna, Tilapia, sardines, mackerel, herring

- Meat – 3-5 oz. grass-fed beef, chicken, turkey, wild turkey, venison, buffalo, or any animal that has never eaten grain contains Omega 3 EPA-DHA, CLA, B 12, and many other B vitamins, iron, zinc, etc.

- Oils – olive oil or coconut oil (2-3 tbs.) as a spread on whole ancient grain bread or use coconut, sesame, grape seed, avocado, or olive oil as a drizzle over fish, salads, rice, potatoes, beans, or other veggies

- Eggs – ideal are cage-free or free-range eggs which contain Omega 3 EPA-DHA along with the variety of fats within. Regular eggs naturally contain monounsaturated, polyunsaturated, and saturated fats in combination, but they do not have Omega 3's.

Note: The Omega 6 grain that chickens and beef are fed, effectively neutralizes any Omega 3 that may have been created within the animal. This is why free-range or grass-fed animals have Omega 3 EPA-DHA, and grain-fed animals do not.

Mix and match 3 servings per day from the above list. According to Dr. Kraus, if you are eating multiple servings of veggies at each meal, especially dark leafy greens and brightly colored veggies as recommended your body will automatically and efficiently metabolize these fats. [16]

Dr. Kraus states that the "body needs a steady supply of proteins and a balance of naturally occurring fats to be healthy." He further points out that saturated fat and cholesterol sources including dairy, coconut, and eggs are fine.

All oils are actually a mix of oils. Olive oil, for instance, is called a monounsaturated fat because the predominant oil, Oleic acid, is monounsaturated. But olive oil also contains some polyunsaturated and saturated fats. Peanut oil and lard contain mostly monounsaturated fats like olive oil, but they also contain some polyunsaturated and saturated fats. Coconut oil and butter contain mostly saturated fats, but they also contain some monounsaturated and polyunsaturated fats. Corn oil, safflower, canola, and soybean oils contain mostly polyunsaturated fats, but they also contain some monounsaturated and saturated fats. [17]   It boils down to the predominance of the type of fatty molecules in the particular food/oil item. Yet, each tablespoon of fat, no matter what kind, has 120 calories, or 9 calories per gram.

Cholesterol

I can hardly talk about fat without bringing up the subject of cholesterol. Did you know that high cholesterol is a sign of *good* health in Japan? Here in the States, at the same time fats were declared to be bad for us, high cholesterol was also deemed to be bad for us. Again, here is inaccurate, incomplete, and selective information. Cholesterol somehow got divided into good and bad. The cholesterol that sticks to the vascular walls is bad; yet, the cholesterol that flows freely is good. This sounds logical, right? This also gave the pharmaceutical companies a reason to come up with statins, which lower cholesterol – bad *and good* cholesterol. In a similar fashion as antibiotics, statins don't choose between bad and good, they wipe out both. But it's not possible to add good cholesterol only, because cholesterol is cholesterol – it divides itself within the body as to how it acts – in reality there is no good and bad. [18]

What does cholesterol do? Your body makes it – on purpose - for several reasons. It acts like a bottle brush and cleans the blood and vascular system. It helps make hormones and helps them function. It enables your body to turn sunshine into the working hormone, vitamin D. It is essential to your body's health! An article by Emil M. deGoma, MD et al. in the *Journal of the American College of Cardiology* posted on Medscape's website describes HDL cholesterol as a powerful anti-inflammatory and antioxidant! [19, 19a]

For those not subscribed to Medscape's excellent medical information, you can find a full medical text and description of HDL's anti-inflammatory and antioxidant properties in *Pharmacological Reviews* titled, "Functionally Defective High-Density Lipoprotein: A New Therapeutic Target at the Crossroads of Dyslipidemia, Inflammation, and Atherosclerosis," by Anatol Kontush and M. John Chapman.

In fact Dr. Mercola states that if your cholesterol gets too low, you may experience bouts of depression, stroke, violent behavior, and even suicide! [20]

Furthermore, researchers at Texas A&M University have discovered that *lower* cholesterol levels can actually *reduce* muscle gain with exercising. [21]

Dr. Harlan Krumholz of the Department of Cardiovascular Medicine at Yale University reported in 1994 that old people with *low* cholesterol died twice as often from a heart attack as did old people with *high* cholesterol. Professor David R. Jacobs and his co-workers from the Division of Epidemiology at the University of Minnesota states that low cholesterol predicted an increased risk of dying from gastrointestinal and respiratory diseases. [22]

If high cholesterol were the most important cause of cardiovascular disease, it should be a risk factor in all populations, in both sexes, at all ages, in all disease categories, and for both heart disease and stroke. But this is not the case.

Uffe Ravnskov, MD, PhD, writes about the "Benefits of High Cholesterol" in an article for Weston Price from his book, *The Cholesterol Myths* (NewTrends Publishing, pp 64-65). "High cholesterol is associated with longevity in old people. It is difficult to explain away the fact that during the period of life in which most cardiovascular disease occurs and from which most people die (and most of us die from cardiovascular disease), high cholesterol occurs most often in people with the lowest mortality. How is it possible that high cholesterol is harmful to the artery walls and causes fatal coronary heart disease, the commonest cause of death, if those whose cholesterol is the highest, live longer than those whose cholesterol is low?" This simply does not compute with what the medical community is telling us. [23]

Coconut oil

Coconut oil is a saturated fat – a plant saturated fat to be specific. As a result, this makes it wholly different than animal saturated fat—in composition, in action, and in health benefits! Coconut oil's predominant saturated fats are a special kind of fatty acids called Medium Chain Triglycerides (MCT's)— the *good* triglycerides which are antibacterial, antimicrobial, antibiotic, antiviral, antifungal, anti-parasitic, anti-carcinogenic, anti-inflammatory and antioxidant!

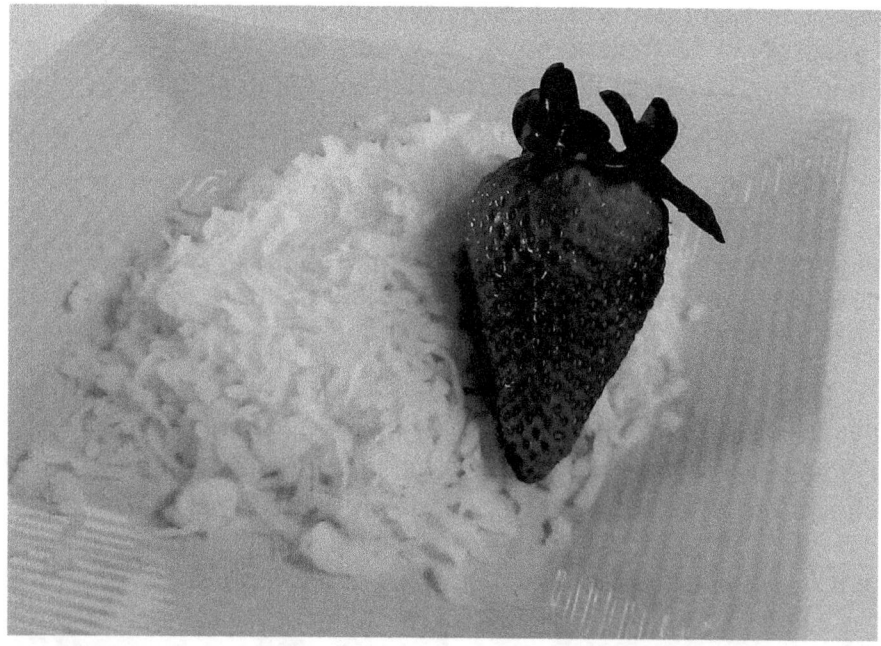

Coconut oil has been used for about four thousand years as *food and medicine* in Polynesian and tropical regions, South and Central America, Africa, the Indian subcontinent and most of Asia. It is not a new thing at all. Yet, when the word "fat," especially "saturated" fat became persona-non-grata in the 1950's, we were inevitably told to kick it to the curb with all the other fats. Unfortunately saturated fats were commonly lumped with hydrogenated and trans fats back then. Nothing could be farther from the truth.

Bruce Fife, ND, CN, explains in his article, "Coconut Oil and Heart Disease," that people in these countries who consume high levels of coconut oil generally have increased levels of HDL (the good cholesterol, which flows freely in your veins) and much better heart health compared to other countries that don't use coconut oil. [24]

Doctor Oz talks about coconut oil, telling us, "…mankind has been consuming mainly saturated fats – in the form of butter, lard, coconut oil, etc. – for thousands of years, yet heart disease was rare before the 1920s. If anything, the rise of heart disease in recent decades may correspond to the increasing use of polyunsaturated vegetable oils like corn, safflower, and canola, as well as margarine." And in regards to obesity and coconut oil, he tells us of the American farmers in the 1940's, who discovered that when they tried to fatten their cattle by feeding them coconut oil, instead of gaining weight, their cattle *lost* weight!" [25]

They lost weight because of the MCTs, which heighten metabolism and increase energy. Unlike other dietary fats which are stored in the body for later use as a backup energy supply, coconut oil goes directly to the liver and is then absorbed and turned into energy. It's not stored as fat by the body, it's used as energy right away! [26]

Coconut oil's MCTs are more easily absorbed than the long or short chain fatty acids, and they even help other nutrients absorb as well. This is why it's so beneficial for those with severe intestinal conditions like Crohn's, Leaky Gut Syndrome, Inflammatory Bowel Disease, Ulcerative Colitis, Candida Albicans, Diverticulitis, and such. These conditions can become deadly when the patient is unable get nutrition into their system no matter how much food they eat. Malnutrition and even starvation is a real threat. [27]

MCTs are rich in Lauric acid, which improves insulin sensitivity and glucose tolerance. Lauric acid has potent antimicrobial properties which helps strengthen the immune system. This is also helpful to give it a long shelf life and help prevent rancidity. [28]

As valuable as coconut oil is for so many conditions, the study I find to be the most impressive, perhaps because it had such a profound effect on my dad is the one which shows its benefits for cognitive function in just one dose! [29]   Sayer Ji's article "MCT Fats Found in Coconut Oil Boost Brain Function in Only One Dose," is nothing short of illuminating! His resources from medical sources are continuing their research, but I find that this food is definitely a healer and have no qualms at all in using it for food *or* medicine!

Oil Pulling

Another way to use coconut oil is Oil Pulling (OP). This is an Ayurvedic treatment, thousands of years old, which is extraordinarily effective not only for oral and dental health— plus whiter teeth, but most importantly as a detoxifier. Removing heavy metals like mercury, lead, cadmium, aluminum and such from your body and brain is extremely important for overall health. In fact, cleansing the mouth, lymph glands and sinuses, can lead to a whole new you!

The process is so simple, yet the therapy has been found to be effective in healing everything from AIDS to diabetes, heart disease to leukemia, sinus infections to allergies, gingivitis to streptococcus infections. [30]

Directions for Oil Pulling:

First thing in the morning, before any food or water has passed your lips, a tablespoon or (heaping teaspoon) of oil is swished around in the mouth and squeezed between the teeth for 5-15 minutes. Then it is spit out into the sink, toilet, or garbage. Do not gargle with it. And *never* swallow the oil after swishing, as it will be *full* of toxins and harmful organisms which you do not want to put back into your body! Sesame, olive, or sunflower oils (unprocessed of course) are also used for OP, but I find the coconut oil has a light, slightly sweet, and pleasant flavor to it. [31]

Even children and babies can release toxins using the oils, by smearing the coconut oil on the soles of the feet then covering with socks at bedtime. Amalgams in the teeth may have mercury and caution is required as these fillings may loosen. Pulling out toxins lets your body know that you are ready to let go of unessential "stuff," and your lower body may want to get in on the act too, loosening and releasing toxins from the other end. [32, 33]

Buying Coconut oil

When buying coconut oil, look for words like organic, expeller pressed, virgin or extra-virgin, and non-refined or non-processed. If you read all these on the label, that's great; but minimally, it should read "organic, virgin coconut oil." I personally prefer the glass container, but plastic is lighter in weight and non-breakable.

I use a lot of it, so I get the larger size, and put some in a smaller container to put in my bedroom for facial and hand cream. I also have a small container of it in my bathroom for zits, mosquito bites or scratches and scrapes. I have another small container in the cat food cabinet for *their* scratches and scrapes! They love the taste, and it heals any of their boo-boo's in a hurry! It also helps when their tummies are not in perfect condition. Coconut oil has even slimmed down my fat cat, Junior!

Olive Oil

Olive oil is the mainstay of the Mediterranean Diet, one of the healthier diets for human beings, which proudly includes lots of veggies and grains, small amounts of meat, sometimes nuts and *generous* portions of olive oil. The fats in olive oil are predominantly monounsaturated. These are the good fats—the healthy fats.

The health benefits of olive oil range from heart health to easing inflammation; from insulin control to bone health; from lowering blood pressure to helping reduce risk of breast cancer; from protecting the liver to protecting against ulcerative colitis and on and on. [34]

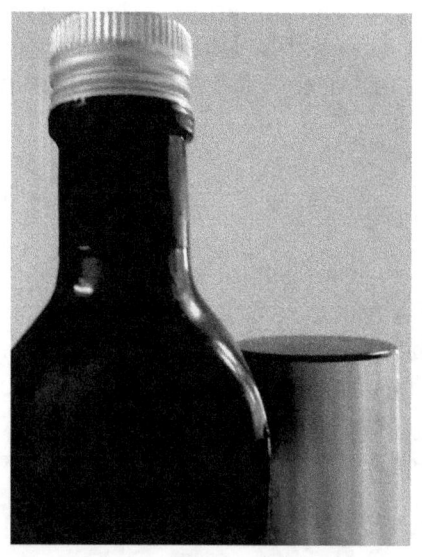

Olive oil comes in many forms – Extra Virgin, Virgin, Pomace (or Pure), and Extra light. Extra Virgin is unrefined and from the first pressing of the choice olives. Virgin oil is also from the first pressing but it has a higher acidity level due to the olives being used or the age of the olives. Pure olive oil is a combination of virgin and refined oils. Extra Light olive oil is *refined* olive oil and is absolutely clear and pale-colored in the bottle. The refinement allows the use of higher heat when used for cooking. However, when it's refined, a lot of the beneficial nutrients are stripped out – flavones, flavonols, lignans, anthocyanidins, etc…the things that give its health benefits. [35]

Smoke Point

When cooking with olive oil, or any oil—vegetable, seed or nut—temperature is a key point to keep in mind – each oil is different. At a specific temperature for each type of oil, the fats begin to break down and start oxidizing – this is called the smoke point. Oxidizing means that free radicals are being formed and a lot of the oil's nutrients are being destroyed. The foods that are now cooked in this oxidized oil absorb those free radicals, and pass them along to you, without any of the oil's benefits. This is why you want to fry in an oil with a high smoke point, which means that it can take a higher heat before it is destroyed or it destroys your food.

Any two bottles of the same oil are slightly different, as the nuts, seeds and olives may be different at the point of origin. So keeping this in mind, the smoke points may vary a bit within the same brand or kind of oil.

The Harvard School of Public Health lists the smoke points for Extra Light (refined) olive oil as 468°F/242°C, and for Extra Virgin (unrefined) olive oil as 320°F/160°C. You can see the difference here. If you want to fry something at a high heat, use the Extra Light refined olive oil. If you want all the health benefits of the oil, it is best to keep the temps lower and use the UN-refined, Extra Virgin olive oil. Or best of all, use the oil as a drizzle on salads or on veggies as a drizzle *after* you've cooked them. [36]

The smoke point of Flaxseed oil 255°F; Coconut oil is 350°F; Grapeseed oil 392°F; Sesame oil 410°F; Sunflower oil 450°F. Avocado oil 520° F. Canola (rapeseed oil) is a *refined* monounsaturated fat with a smoke point of 400°F. For a list of more vegetable, nut, and seed oil's smoke points see *What's Cooking America* website. [37]

Buying olive oil

According to Dr. Donald Hensrud of the Mayo Clinic, care must be taken with olive oil; because, just like bottled/liquid Omega 3 fish oils—heat, light, and air can break down the oils; and, it can become oxidized right there in the bottle by any or all three repeated exposures over a minimum period of time. The oil should be stored in a dark room-temperature cupboard, or even the refrigerator. The healthy fats and phytonutrients slowly degrade over time as well, so if it's been opened at all, it's best to use it up within four to six months, and if kept properly, maybe up to a year. If the taste or aroma becomes bitter or rancid, toss it! [38] It is also best to purchase oils in a dark colored glass container as this helps keep the light out.

Also, beware of counterfeit olive oil. It's become a very big business. According to *Consumer Reports* (CR), the "Extra Virgin" olive oil is carefully screened, meeting exacting standards in Europe. But the standards in the U.S. are not nearly as stringent and much of what is passed along to us is completely subpar! In 2012, CR tests showed that 23 Extra Virgin olive oils were badly flawed and not worthy of the label! Some are even mixed with sunflower or safflower oil. At the price of good olive oil, you want the real deal – no mixtures or substitutes! [39]

A National Public Radio.com article by Allison Aubrey in September 2013, tells that more than half of the Extra

Virgin olive oil imported into the U.S. has been found to be substandard. It's such a low-grade oil that it doesn't give the health benefits or even have the taste that Extra Virgin should give you. Sometimes it's a simple case of the oil being too old, or being improperly stored in a warm warehouse before being shipped. [40]

A study from the University of California, Davis, found that 69% of imports tested failed to meet a U.S Department of Agriculture quality standard. [41]

Mark Sisson of Mark's Daily Apple.com, gives a few examples of how to check for quality. [42]   One way to see if your olive oil is not a mixture of other oils, is to put it in the refrigerator and see if it solidifies. The oleic acid (the predominant monounsaturates in the oil) will solidify at 39°. This of course means that you must buy it first to find out. But even that is not a sure way to tell because some companies have come up with some pretty good substitutes as *Consumer Reports* has found out.

The moral of this story is whenever possible purchase local, freshly made olive oil. Best yet, make your own! Check a recent issue of *Consumer Reports* to find out which oils have passed muster this current year. Maybe check out your local Italian restaurants and see what they use. Test and try to find one you trust, and stick with that brand. Check and see if there is a date stamped on it – the date the olives were pressed or the expiration date. The effort is definitely worth it for the health benefits!

Avocados

Also called the "alligator pear" due to its appearance, the avocado is one of the healthiest foods around. Some call it a super food or a perfect food, on a par with the apple. One avocado packs a whopping 4 grams of protein – good protein too, with 18 of the most important amino acids. An average avocado contains twice as much potassium as a banana,

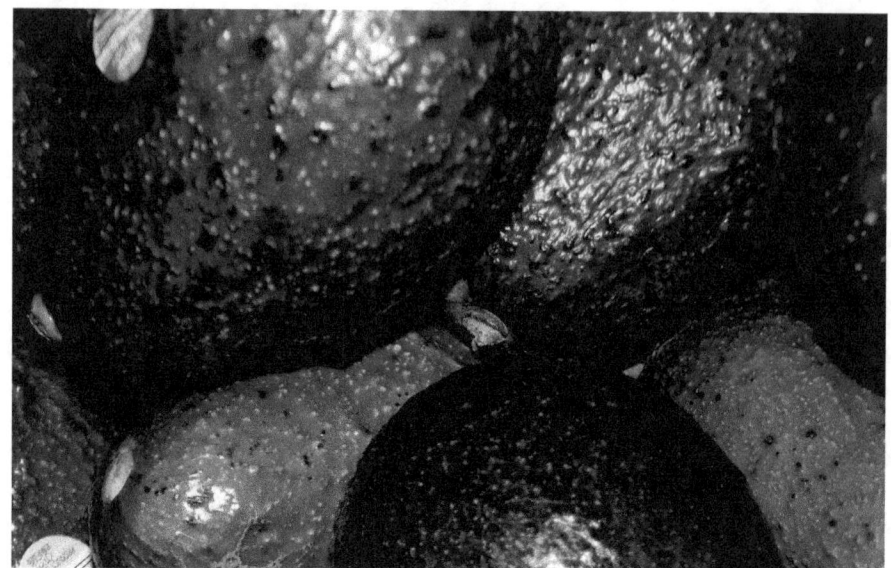

healthy monounsaturated fats, which include a large portion of healthy oleic acid found in olive oil—Omega 3 ALA, loads of fiber, magnesium, B-vitamins, Folic Acid, vitamins E, C, and K. Avocados actually have more than 20 essential health-boosting nutrients!

Important note: For those with a Latex allergy, this fruit is NOT for you. Like bananas and chestnuts, avocados have a high amount of chitinase enzymes which would activate this allergy, causing chronic throat clearing and sinus issues and/ or other very serious conditions. Cooking may deactivate these enzymes, but for safety sake, treat it with caution!

According to Dr. Mercola, who eats an avocado every day, it is one of the fruits (yes, it's a fruit, not a vegetable) that can be safe even if non-organic, due to its tough hide! Pesticides can't seem to penetrate it. [43]

Although avocados are heavy in calories, they are nutrient dense with healthy fat calories and are listed very low on the glycemic index. [44] In fact, according to a new study published

Pati Chandler

in *Nutrition Journal*, they discovered that avocado eaters had a lower than average weight, smaller waistline and a lower BMI than non-consumers! [45]

Yet, that's only the tip of the iceberg here. A research team at the University of California published a study in the journal, *Food and Nutrition* providing evidence that consuming half a fresh avocado on a burger significantly inhibited the production of the inflammatory compound IL-6, compared to eating a burger without the avocado. What this means is that the slice of avocado virtually stopped the inflammatory response of the grilled burger! [46]

This leathery fruit has wide-ranging health benefits, including benefits for the brain, the heart, eyes, blood pressure, blood sugar, digestion, free radical damage, and pregnancy, due to its high amount of folic acid, plus B-vitamins and healthy fats. Avocados are anti-inflammatory and full of enzymes and antioxidants, particularly glutathione, the master antioxidant. It also helps your body make even more glutathione – giving it a boost, as it were. Glutathione cleans up and recycles other "used" antioxidants like vitamins A, C, and E, and puts them back to work! Glutathione supports the liver and the nervous system and helps boost the immune system. [47]

With its high concentration of phytochemicals, the anti-inflammatory and antioxidant factors, the avocado has been shown to help prevent cancers of the mouth, skin, breast, and prostate gland. [48]

George Mateljan, author, nutritionist, researcher, and originator of the website, *The World's Healthiest Foods*, tells us, "One cup of fresh avocado (150 grams) added to a salad of romaine lettuce, spinach, and carrots increased absorption of carotenoids from this salad between 200-400%. This research result makes perfect sense to us because carotenoids are fat-soluble and would be provided with the fat they need for absorption from the addition of avocado. Avocado oil added to a salad accomplished this same result. Interestingly, both avocado oil and fresh avocado added to salsa increased carotenoid absorption from the salsa as well." [49]

Avocado oil has a high smoke point of 520° so it is quite an excellent oil for stir fry or browning, and it's delicious as a delightful drizzle on salad with many of the above mentioned health benefits.

To learn ways to use avocados in your daily diet, there are approximately 911 recipes available on the *Food Network* alone! [50] You can also type in your search engine "Avocado Recipes" and get hundreds more!

TIP ONE When shopping for avocados, choose a firm, not hard, or too soft a fruit, with no dark sunken spots or cracks. If you choose a firmer fruit, you can ripen it at home in a paper bag or in a fruit basket within a few days. Use the "nick and peel" method to open an avocado. Most of the best nutrients are found in the dark outer layer, just under its leathery hide. So the idea is *not* to throw that way with the skin. Start by slicing it in half lengthwise, then going around the seed.

TIP TWO Avocados and avocado oil are most beneficial on the outside too! The avocado and avocado oil are excellent skin conditioners and are widely used in the cosmetics industry. With its natural vitamins, minerals, antioxidants and healthy natural oils, it is an excellent moisturizer and eye cream, especially used at night. It's wonderful on knees, elbows, heels and calluses.

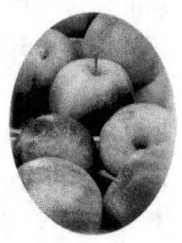

Chapter 5

Carbohydrates

Carbohydrates include fiber, starches, and sugars. The sugars and starches are used by your body to make glucose, which is fuel for the body (aka energy) especially for the brain and nervous system. [1]   This glucose can either be used immediately or stored – in the liver or muscles.

As the "plate" in Fig 2 describes carbohydrates (carbs) should consist of about 50% of your meal; and the bulk, if not all of this 50%, would ideally be complex carbs.

Technically speaking, everything except pure fat, plain meat, and finned fish (that eat other fish) are the only foods that do NOT have carbohydrates in them. Phytoplankton and algae, which many fish eat, have carbohydrates and are then passed into the meat of the fish, which we eat. Cows that eat grain, are eating carbohydrates, and again are passed along to us in their meat or their milk and other dairy. [2]

This brings us to the types of carbs that are available to us, simple and complex as they are. Within these two types are yet more subdivisions, but I won't bog you down with details. Simple carbohydrates are digested and absorbed very quickly. Complex carbohydrates take their time being digested and absorbed. Fiber is a member of the complex carb family and isn't absorbed at all, but it's still absolutely necessary to our health, as discussed in the upcoming section on "Prebiotics."

Simple Carbohydrates

Simple carbohydrates that contain natural healthy vitamins and minerals include fruits, milk and vegetables, but also *raw* honey, raw agave, raw maple syrup and raw molasses – raw, meaning unrefined, heated, or processed. These latter four just happen to have more calories, so moderation is in order. Although considered foods in their raw state due to the high vitamin, mineral and enzyme content, they should be used more or less as condiments. "The whites" are included in this simple sugar category – *refined* white bread, rice, and pasta.

All simple carbohydrates digest and absorb at warp speed, raising blood sugar quickly, especially when eaten alone without protein, fats, or complex carbs.

Simple carbohydrates include:

- Fructose - fruits

- Galactose - milk

- Lactose - milk and dairy

- Maltose - some vegetables and beer

- Sucrose - table sugar, corn syrup

- Foods with added sugars such as jams, fruit drinks, cereal, cookies, donuts, crackers, ketchup, salad dressings, soft drinks etc. utilize all of the above "ose" simple sugars and more.

Complex Carbohydrates

Carbohydrates are in all foods derived from plants. All

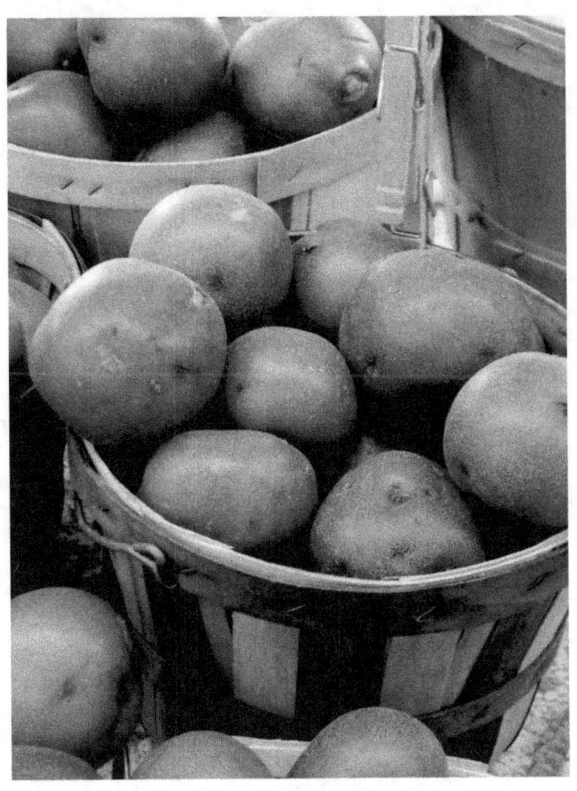

complex carbohydrates are nutrient rich and filled with vitamins, minerals, and enzymes, along with fiber and/or starches. These carbs come in linked chains of three or more sugar molecules, and are much slower to digest and absorb than the simple carbohydrates because of their molecular complexity. This helps the blood sugar to stay more even and prevent spikes in blood sugar readings. They also help balance out protein and fat absorption in an even manner.

Complex carbs consist of fiber, starch, and sugars...slow sugars – complex sugars. The starches and sugars are energy sources, and the fiber is a digestive aid, which also happens to help prevent diseases, especially those of the digestive system like Crohn's, Diverticulitis, irritable bowel issues, and so on.

Complex Carbohydrates include:

- Vegetables

- Starchy vegetables – peas, beans, corn, potatoes*

- Legumes

- Nuts

- Seeds

- *Whole* grains**- quinoa, whole grain barley, whole grain oats, buckwheat, bulgur, wild rice, brown rice, popcorn [3,4]

> **Basically, foods that grow are the best carbohydrates for our body.**

Fiber

Dietary fiber, also known as roughage or bulk, is included in the complex carb category and includes all the parts of plant foods that the enzymes in your body can't digest or absorb. It comes in soluble and insoluble forms as described in the section on "Prebiotics." Unfortunately, foods high in fiber are generally not common on the average plate. According to the CDC (Centers for Disease Control), we need 28-35 grams of fiber each day, and we aren't getting it. [5]

One apple a day doesn't do it. One order of whole grain toast doesn't do it. One potato doesn't do it. Try adding a whole fiber food at each meal. And snack on a fiber food in between meals – apple, pear, figs, berries, nuts, humus, popcorn, sunflower seeds, etc. It's filling and healing at the same time. It also keeps things moving along exceptionally well.

Refined grain fiber, such as "the whites"—white breads, biscuits, donuts, pastries, pizza, pasta, white rice, and the like, have been processed to death and have little or no fiber left, much less vitamins and minerals. When you see words like "refined," "enriched" or "fortified" you know that nearly all the good stuff has been taken out in the processing, and then man-made folic acid, vitamin C, Iron, and the like, have been added back into it...because we need it. Yet, it's not quite the same thing as the "real thing" that Mother Nature put in there, where all the right amounts of the right stuff work together for our benefit.

Bentley Thompson is an engineering consultant, but he's also a medical author of numerous articles on diabetes, and the author of *The 7 Biggest Mistakes in Your Diet and How to Avoid Them* (a seven part e-mail mini-course). He is also the owner of the excellent diabetic website *DiabeticCarbGuide. com* where he states, "When high fiber complex carbohydrate foods make up 75% of calories per meal the results have been tremendous." He tells that this type of diet has caused many diabetics to discontinue their medication and insulin in a very short time. He also tells us that researchers have shown for long term use and effectiveness, diet proportions illustrated in the "plate" in Fig. 2 may provide the optimum diet for diabetics. 6

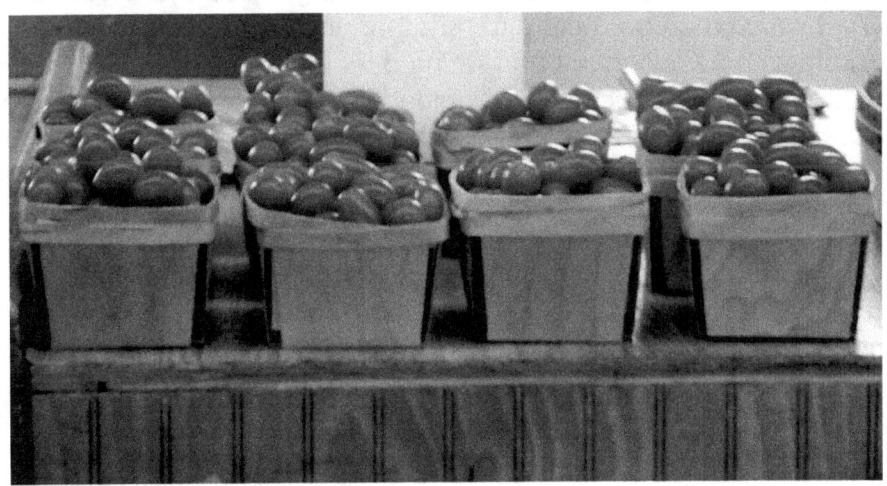

A nice little side effect of high fiber foods is that they tend to be foods that are also *high* in antioxidants and *low* in fat and calories! Examples are in the skins of many foods where the fiber is surrounding the foods as well as on the inside like apples, pears, tomatoes, grapes, potatoes, and so on.

If you have been low in fiber, and are intending to increase your intake, build up slowly and be sure to drink a lot of water. This helps move the fiber along to do its job.

Glycemic Index

The Glycemic Index is a numerical index that ranks carbohydrates based on their rate of conversion to glucose (sugar) in the body – the glycemic response. Or more simply, it tells how fast the food will raise your blood sugar—the lower the number on this Index, the better, *and slower* the conversion to glucose. In general, foods in the complex group are low on the glycemic index and foods in the simple carb group are rated as high. There are numerous exceptions though, so if one intends to use the Glycemic Index as a guide for their food choice, a chart would be necessary to be accurate.

Foods rated below 50 are the ideal, even though the foods that are a bit over 50 are *periodically* acceptable. It can get complicated though, because of something called the Glycemic Load which may be quite different than the actual index. Foods with a Glycemic Load rating over 20 are considered to be undesirable, especially for diabetics. This load takes into account not only the Index rating but the nutrient advantage and serving size too. A food with a high Index rating can sometimes have a low Load rating; this is where the charts come in handy. [7]

Both of these indices are handy for those with diabetes, hypoglycemia, or Metabolic Syndrome or even those on a diet, because it can help guide food choices in order to help stabilize blood sugar. Harvard Medical School has a list of 100 foods in their Glycemic Index and Glycemic Load located in their website. [8]

According to their chart, an average apple on their list has a glycemic index of 39, and a glycemic load of 6. Safe and healthy to be sure. Kidney beans have an Index number of 29 and a Load number of 7. Also good. Regular white spaghetti noodles—Index at 58, Load at 26. *Not* good. Boiled white potatoes – Index at 82, and Load at 21—also not good. These latter two are obviously high, all the way around. But when you add protein and fat, it helps balance out a *small* portion of these food items and they become more acceptable.

According to Sandra Meyerowitz, MPH, RD, a nutritionist and owner of *Nutrition Works* in Louisville, KY, "It makes more sense to use the glycemic load because when you eat a food, you don't just eat one food by itself — you eat a whole bunch of foods together. Looking at the total picture of foods you eat, rather than just the individual pieces, gives you a clearer and more accurate picture of the foods that make up your diet." [9]

The idea to take away here is that there are carbs and then there are healthy, beneficial, and essential carbs. A low carb diet may be detrimental to your health, especially if you are cutting out the complex carbs and fibers you need to maintain a healthy body. This is especially important when it comes to antioxidants.

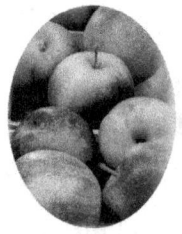

Chapter 6

Antioxidants

Everyone has heard about antioxidants and most people understand that they are a good thing, even if they don't exactly know why. Antioxidants neutralize and "disarm" free radicals. What are free radicals? Free radicals are highly excited and unstable molecules that are created in your body by normal metabolic functions. Yet, in this 21st century we are *also* bombarded by free radicals that we never saw coming 100 years ago. A googolplex of free radicals also come at us on a daily, hourly, even minute-to-minute basis, from this modern environment and from the modern harsh foods we eat.

In our bodies, free radicals are literally the waste products of successful cellular transactions. Nutrients, oxygen, and catalysts (Magnesium, Calcium, CoQ10, Malate, etc.) enter the cell, and through their magical process become a unit of energy called Adenosine Triphosphate (ATP). The waste products from these transactions are often free radicals. Prolonged, regular use of the necessary Omega 3 fish oil also creates free radicals. This is perfectly normal, and a healthy body is equipped with *free radical scavengers* that disarm and neutralize these radicals regularly throughout the day. These scavengers (antioxidants) are natural chemicals in the body such as certain enzymes and antioxidants like Alpha Lipoic Acid (ALA), CoQ10, Glutathione, and Superoxide Dismutase (SOD), catalase (CAT), peroxidase enzymes, and melatonin.

The antioxidants that we *eat* are boosters to our own, internally-made antioxidants. But we also get a plethora of different antioxidants from foods, like vitamins A, C, E, and selenium (the ACES), resveratrol, polyphenols, flavonoids, carotenoids, countless phytochemicals, etc! And what foods do we get them from?

Antioxidants are found in:

- Fruits

- Vegetables

- Starchy vegetables – peas, beans, corn, potatoes

- Legumes

- Nuts

- Seeds

- Whole grains

Does this list look familiar? It should. It's the same list as complex carbohydrates, with fruit added! All these foods boost our body's ability to make its own antioxidants, while at the same time adding even more antioxidants to our system from the foods themselves.

According to WebMD.com all fruits and veggies contain antioxidants, but the ones containing the most are: apples, berries, peaches, mangos, melons, beans, russet potatoes, sweet potatoes, spinach, artichoke hearts and eggplant. [1]
And look for foods of color - dark greens, reds, purples and oranges…even dark brown, as in dark chocolate!

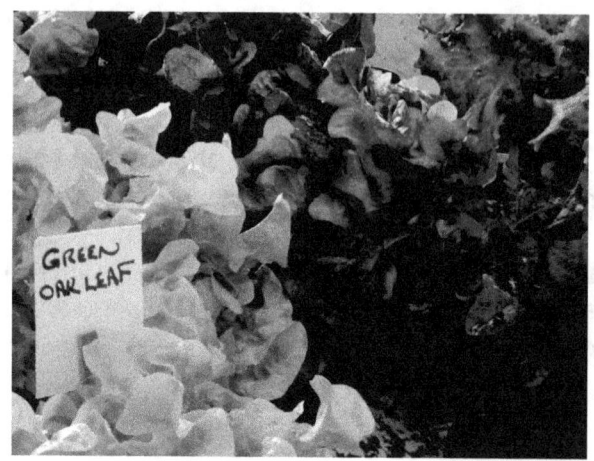

We need to eat food daily of course, because we use up the nutrients daily as fuel. But when we keep adding inflammatory foods to our bodies, we are making more and more free radicals – fried foods, hydrogenates, sugar, artificial sweeteners, and all the rest. They produce inflammation by adding free radicals! That's why it is imperative that we add antioxidants to neutralize them.

The *Harvard School of Public Health* recommends 5-13 servings of fruits and veggies per day. [2] Because we do have control over what we eat, we can control some of the free radicals that are greatly affecting our body. Imagine how effective these antioxidants would be if we didn't eat those harsh foods in the first place.

If our enzyme stores are low, as is often the case in a chronically ill body, and if our body has begun to slow down in its manufacturing of natural antioxidants like ALA, CoQ10, melatonin, and the like—and if we don't faithfully eat 5 to 13 servings, *or more*, of fruits and veggies, nuts and grains every single day, then… well, we are going to have an overabundance of free radicals running amok in our body, frantically looking to latch onto something they shouldn't in order to stabilize themselves. This can create a whole host of problems starting with inflammation and ending with a chronic illness like Alzheimer's, muscular sclerosis, diabetes, cancer, chronic fatigue, and so much more!

Then there are the free radicals that enter our body, unbidden, from the environment—exposure to radiation, X-rays, cigarette smoke, electromagnetic fields (EMFs), household and industrial chemicals, air pollution, auto exhaust, pesticides, herbicides, and more. Antioxidants help us here too. Often these are things we just can't get away from, but adding a generous supply of antioxidants daily can help neutralize these unwanted and unbidden free radicals.

Free Radicals

When you slice an apple, the surface turns brown. The layer of cells that are brown have died. This is oxidation. When you get a cut on your finger, the cells at the edges of that cut oxidize and die, while the blood clots to seal the wound. Your body then begins to replace the old dead cells with new cells. [3]

The apple is no longer able to repair itself once it's plucked off the tree so, it cannot replace the dead cells with living cells. In our case, if our immune system is up to par, our body can heal that cut with no problem, in just a few days. But if our immune system is compromised by too many free radicals, poor nutrition, chronic illness, or what have you, it will take a really long time for your body to repair that cut. It may even become infected before it gets repaired. Antioxidants help boost the immune system and decrease inflammation, helping this repair work.

Free radicals destroy protective cell membranes. They latch onto the cells' membranes to try and stabilize themselves, and end up destroying parts of the cell or even killing them. Most importantly, these free radicals damage the all-important DNA within the cells. So now, when this damaged DNA replicates, it actually duplicates a damaged cell! And these new irregular damaged cells seem to grow like a California wildfire!

This cell damage also greatly compromises and impairs the immune system, leading to all kinds of infections and any number of chronic and degenerative diseases as these damaged cells duplicate over and over. Free radicals make inflammation in the process of this rapid growth, creating mayhem unlike anything we ever want in our bodies! Uncontrolled growth such as this is also characteristic of cancer cells.

What Do Antioxidants Do?

Antioxidants prevent and reverse this damage to cells. Because antioxidants are specialists, different antioxidants will work in different areas of the body. But all in all, they neutralize free radicals by either interrupting their process or by binding with them and unceremoniously escorting them OUT of our body...*before* they latch onto something. It is believed by some that addressing this free radical issue is a vital part of helping many factors in nearly *all* chronic and degenerative diseases, including fibromyalgia, Chronic Fatigue Syndrome, rheumatoid arthritis, muscular sclerosis, heart disease, and cancer.

Antioxidants benefit us in 3 basic ways:

1. They help relieve pain and inflammation by getting rid of excess free radicals – either by neutralizing, interrupting, or preventing them from materializing in the first place.
2. They are extremely beneficial immune system boosters.
3. Most foods that contain antioxidants are also alkaline in pH, and so they help neutralize acids in your body.

Antioxidants work synergistically. That is, they work better together than alone. Because antioxidants specialize, each working specifically in one or two areas in the body, it is better to take a moderate amount of several different kinds of antioxidants rather than a *lot* of any *one* antioxidant. Too much vitamin A, for example can be toxic. Too much vitamin E can affect diabetes, thyroid, and heart issues.

> *It is better to take a moderate amount of several different kinds of antioxidants*
>
> *rather than an excessive amount of any one antioxidant.*

Taking antioxidants regularly throughout the day, every day is highly recommended. Taking extra antioxidants is wise even if you really DO eat up to 13 servings of fruit and veggies per day. With a chronically ill body making free radicals at a supersonic pace, and being constantly bombarded from the outside with them, it's an excellent idea to get all the antioxidants you can on a regular—*daily*—basis.

Buying Antioxidant Supplements

Some antioxidants that are available in supplement form are: Alpha Lipoic Acid, vitamins A, C, E, Selenium, Beta-carotene, Bilberry, Burdock, CoQ10, GABA (Gama-AminoButyric acid), Garlic, Ginkgo, Glutathione, Grape Seed

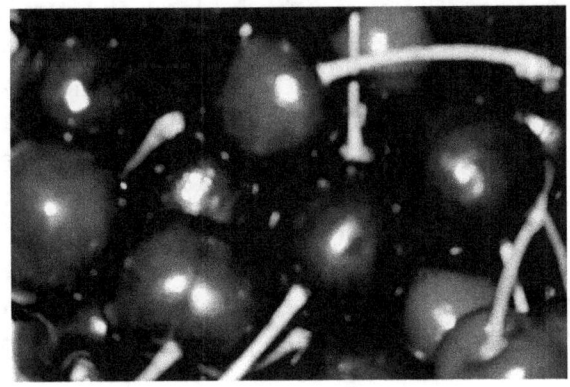

Extract, Green Tea, Melatonin, NADH (Nicotinamide adenine dinucleotide), Quercetin, Turmeric, and Zinc.

All fresh fruits, vegetables, nuts, whole grains, and legumes have plenty of antioxidants—flavonoids, polyphenols and resveratrol, and phytochemicals for example. So foods are the best source of course! Especially as they also have fiber, vitamins, minerals, enzymes, and the like on the inside!

Other antioxidants introduced to the market recently are Açai Juice, Mangostene Juice, Noni Juice, Goji Juice, and Pomegranate Juice. Here again each one is work specific, so a bit of each one works better than a lot of any particular one.

Although not exactly new to the market, there are two exceptional antioxidant products available. The popular Juice Plus+® product is a combination of more than a dozen fruits or vegetables or berries, depending on the capsules taken, and Xocai® Chocolate is a chocolate product with an exceptional amount of antioxidants, combining Cacao and Açai in the confection. Both are loaded with a combination of antioxidants.

7 TIPS

1. Tart cherries, tart cherry juice, dried tart cherries or even the tart cherry supplement are all very high in antioxidants. They have the added benefit of being a Cox2 inhibitor – a natural pain reliever that man tries to create and put into some pain relievers. In fact, nothing works better than tart cherries to relieve painful gout. Five to eight dried tart cherries, or a shot glass of the juice two or three times a day can do wonders for arthritis or muscle pain! And because they contain melatonin, they even help you get to sleep, and *stay* asleep, later in the evening when you're ready, while helping you stay calm and

relaxed during the day. [4]

2. Turmeric, the spice, is also a supremely potent antioxidant that has the powerful pain reliever curcumin as its active ingredient. This is the part that does the pain relieving, inflammation fighting, and immune boosting. It is also the part that can kill cancer cells! Turmeric boosts your own antioxidants, glutathione, catalase, and superoxide dismutase. [5] The Turmeric root can be ground and sprinkled into pot stews, on eggs, salads, sauces, green smoothies—whatever! You might consider adding a bit of black pepper with it, as its main alkaloid, piperine, can increases the absorption of the curcumin. [6] Actually this piperine can increase the absorption of many nutrients found in foods, so feel free to sprinkle pepper on just about everything. Turmeric can also be purchased in capsule form, but be certain the capsule contains at least 95% curcuminoids. Therapeutic doses under medical supervision ranges from 5,000-8,000 mg (5-8 grams) per day, but 600-2,000 mg are quite sufficient for starters.

3. Holy Basil, also called Tulsi, is an herb with very

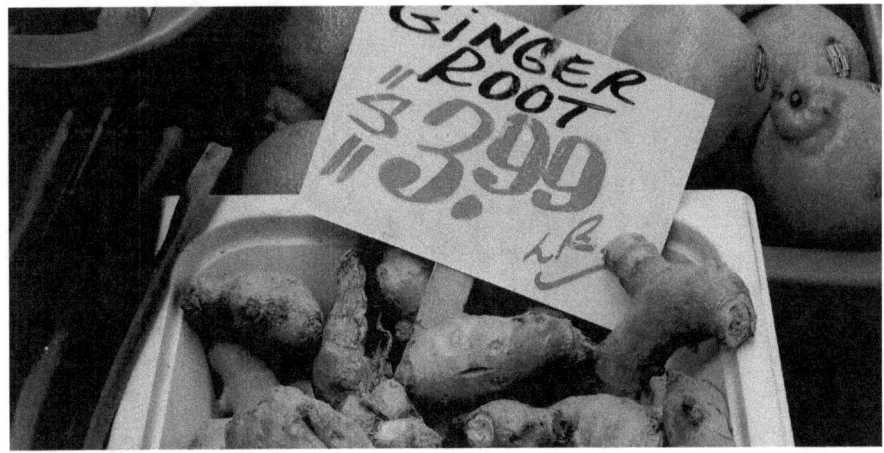

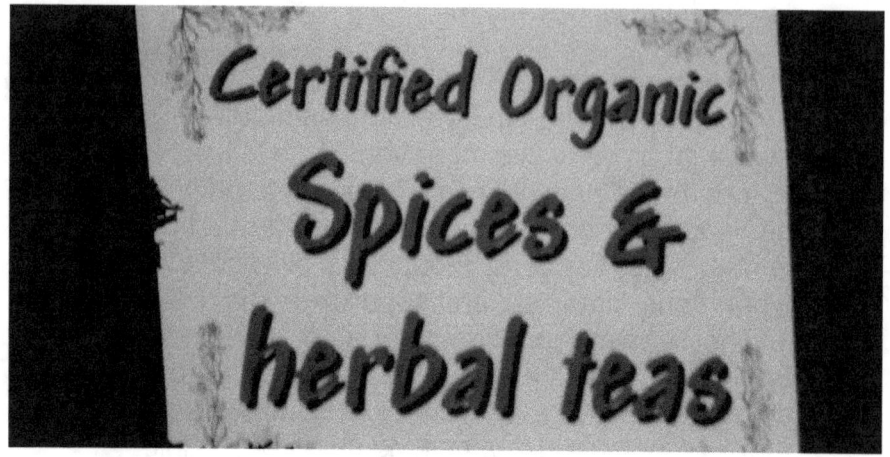

potent antioxidants. Sweet basil, the cooking herb, also has many antioxidants, although it is milder in action. The Holy Basil plant has been used for centuries as an adaptogen, helping to ease stress and balance hormones and mood, while boosting energy at the same time. It is anti-bacterial, anti-fungal, and anti-inflammatory.[7] Tulsi is a delicious tea all by itself, but the popular company Organic India® makes it in many flavors: Pomegranate Green, Sweet Rose, Jasmine, Lemon Ginger, Green, Raspberry Peach, Vanilla Crème, and so on.

4. Green tea is full of antioxidants, especially EGCG (epigallocatechin gallate). This is a very special flavonoid which has been proven to help treat many types of cancers, cardiovascular disease, diabetes, obesity, Alzheimer's, Parkinson's disease, and more. [8] Five cups or more of organic green tea per day were generally used in studies, but the green tea extract (capsule) was used as well. Of course, there have been studies going on for thousands of years in the Orient, so they already know the value of this potent healthy drink. L-Theanine, an amino acid, is a major bonus found in green tea. L-Theanine has

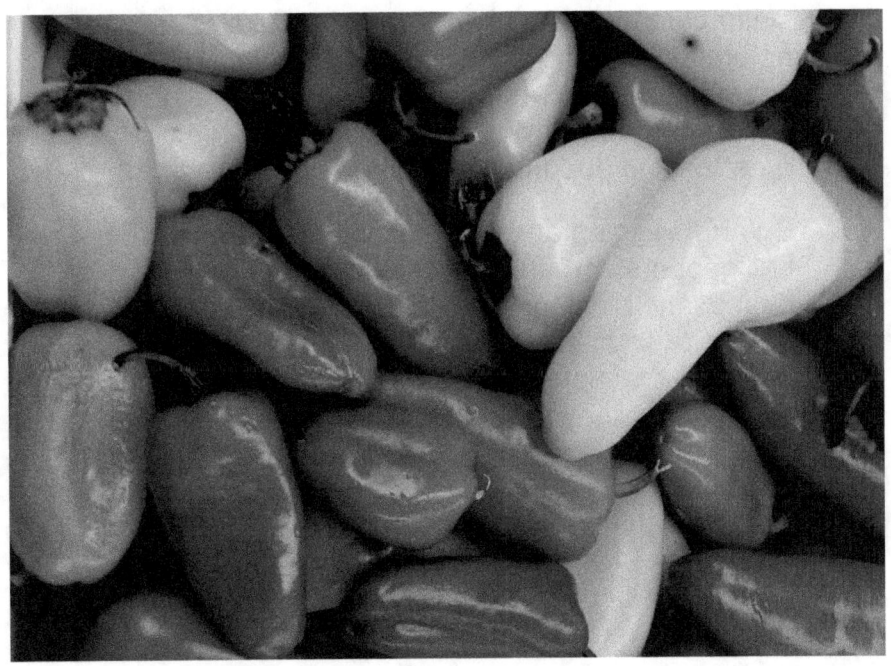

a chemical structure very similar to glutamine, and both neurotransmitters that come from it, and it works in a very similar fashion by helping to transmit nerve impulses. This helps focus and concentration by allowing the brain to relax and concentrate without making you sleepy. Yet at the same time, it can relax the brain so that sleep *can* be enhanced. It's not a sedative, but a balancer which calms the mind. [9] Indeed it is an ingredient in a number of over-the-counter sleep aids.

5. Ginger, the spice, is also a powerful antioxidant and a potent pain reliever. It is most especially used for easing stomach issues, but it is also a potent anti-inflammatory, pain-reliever and immune booster.

6. Garlic and onions are powerful antioxidants with superior immune system boosters. The powerful

sulfur compound inside helps make them excellent natural antibiotic, antibacterial, and anti-inflammatory vegetables. They are good for the heart and good for circulation. Aside from all these benefits, they taste great adding good flavor to any meal or stew!

7. Colorful veggies and legumes like beets, eggplant, bell peppers, tomatoes, kidney beans, small red beans, and black beans are all excellent antioxidants. The color says it all. The deeper, richer, and darker the color the more flavones, phytonutrients, and antioxidants they have!

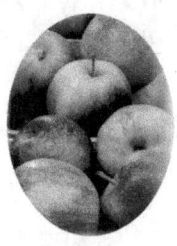

Epilogue

"If you always do what you've always done, you'll always get what you've always gotten."

~Modernization of a quote by Lao Tsu.

The human body was made to heal itself, which it can and does do when it is given the proper nutrition and assistance to do so.

Proteins, fats and carbohydrates provide all the nutrients our body needs to promote growth, maintenance and repair on a daily basis. Anything that does *not* promote growth of healthy cells, provide daily maintenance or cellular repair is unnecessary and most likely a primary factor in leading to, developing and maintaining a chronic condition.

Because inflammation is the most basic factor in all chronic and/or autoimmune conditions, our first line of defense is to eliminate as much inflammation as we possibly can. When these inflammatory cytokines are blocking and otherwise interfering with our body's internal communication systems, we must get to the source in order to give ourselves a fighting chance.

Taking care of *symptoms* caused by the inflammation is not effective in the long run, and may even be counterproductive. The idea is to get to the cause – the inflammation – and neutralize that.

We can help get to the root of the problem by implementing this 3-Step program:

1) Stop feeding the fire and eliminate or severely cut back on inflammatory foods

2) Bring back the balance necessary for your body to have a fighting chance

3) Start putting out the fire with healthy, nutritious, and *healing* foods.

Continually adding inflammatory and acidic foods can UNDO all your best efforts in attempting to ease symptoms and heal. All the good supplements, antioxidants, healthy foods, even, acupuncture, or chiropractic work has no chance of any long-lasting results if we continually add fuel to the fire. Taking these healthy antioxidants for example, followed by a bag of French fries and/or a can of pop cancels out the antioxidants. It's like a plus and a minus canceling each other out, except in this case the *minus* has the upper hand, and the inflammation proves it!

When these harsh foods are eaten as a "treat" once or twice a month, there may not be much of an effect on a chronically ill body. But on a daily, or three-times-a-day, basis...well, you can see where your body has no chance to "catch up."

Foods that have been processed, hydrogenated, and generally stripped of all healthy nutrition is *not* in our best interest, even if they have been "fortified," and "enriched" with man-made folic acid, vitamin C, or anything else.

Whole, rich, natural, *real* foods are healing foods. They come complete, the way they were intended to be—with fiber, vitamins, minerals, amino acids, natural fatty acids, enzymes and probiotics. These are foods that can help your pain and potentially even heal your body.

> *Food can cure or create disease...the trick is to learn which food does what!*

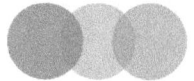

Author Bio

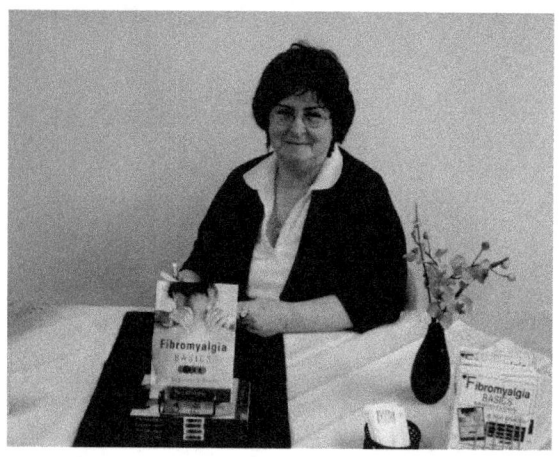

Pati Chandler was diagnosed with Arthritis in 1990, Ankylosing Spondylitis in 1995, and fibromyalgia in 1998. It was the fibromyalgia that urged her to research natural options. It became quickly evident that prescriptions weren't getting her where she wanted to be, healthwise. So as she researched, tested and tried a variety of supplements, alternative treatments and foods, she found the "right combination" for her and never looked back. Her last doctor visit for symptoms of these conditions was in the year 2000. Choosing the right foods and natural options has helped all her symptoms to where she leads a normal life, free of daily pain; even the flares are short-lived and manageable.

Chandler is currently the mother of four, grandmother of six, and great-grandmother of one. She is a nature-lover and rock-hound who enjoys playing with her two cats, watching "feel-good" movies and listening to books-on-CD, because it leaves her hands free to do other things!

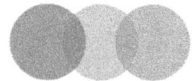

References

Introduction
Preface

1. University of Maryland Medical Journal. *Mind-body medicine.* October 2, 2011. http://www.umm.edu/altmed/articles/mind-body-000355.htm. Accessed Jan. 22, 2014.
2. Bair, M J, Robinson, R L, Katon W, Kroenke K. *Depression and Pain Comorbidity: A Literature Review.* NCBI PubLmEd.gov. November 2003. http://www.ncbi.nlm.nih.gov/pubmed/14609780 Accessed Jan. 22, 2014.
3. Marten, Sylvia. *How Chronic Pain Leads to Depression.* Spine-Health.com. February 21, 2008. http://www.spine-health.com/blog/how-chronic-pain-leads-depression Accessed Jan. 22, 2014.
4. University of Maryland Medical Center. http://www.umm.edu/altmed/articles/mind-body-000355.htm Accessed Jan. 22, 2014.

Part 1, Step One: Stop Feeding the Fire
Chapter 1 – A Few Words about Inflammation

1. Arizona Center for Advanced Medicine, Chronic Inflammation. http://arizonaadvancedmedicine.com/chronic-inflammation/ Accessed Jan. 22, 2014.
2. Arizona Center for Advanced Medicine, Chronic Inflammation. http://arizonaadvancedmedicine.com/chronic-inflammation/ Accessed Jan. 22, 2014.

3. Mercola DO, Joseph M. *Americans are Less Healthy, and Die Sooner than People in other Developed Nations.* Mercola.com. January 23, 2013. http://articles.mercola.com/sites/articles/archive/2013/01/23/united-states-health-ranking.aspx Accessed Jan. 22, 2014.

4. *Inflammation: The Secret Leading Cause of Disease and What to Do About It,* Heavy Metal Detox, 2013, http://articles.healthrealizations.com/HeavyMetalDetox/2013/09/30/Inflammation-The-Secret-Leading-Cause-of.aspx?SubscriberEmail=ianclements%40hotmail.com Accessed Jan. 22, 2014.

Chapter 2 – Stop Feeding the Fire

1. WebMD.com. *What's an Elimination Diet?* November 13, 2012. http://www.webmd.com/allergies/guide/allergies-elimination-diet Accessed Jan. 22, 2014.

2. Appleton, Nancy. *141 Reasons Sugar Ruins Your Health.* Nancyappleton.com http://nancyappleton.com/141-reasons-sugar-ruins-your-health/ Accessed Jan. 22, 2014.

3. Thedoctorwithin.com, http://www.thedoctorwithin.com/minerals/minerals/ Accessed Jan. 29, 2014.

4. Mike. *The Health Effects of Drinking Soda - Quotes from the Experts.* Naturalnews.com. January 08, 2005. http://www.naturalnews.com/004416_soft_drinks_osteoporosis.html Accessed Jan. 22, 2014.

5. American Heart Association. *Sugars and Carbohydrates.* June 11, 2012. http://www.heart.org/HEARTORG/GettingHealthy/NutritionCenter/HealthyDietGoals/Sugars-and-Carbohydrates_UCM_303296_Article.jsp Accessed Jan. 22, 2014.

6. Whole Raw Food Now. *Diet Soda Dilemma.* January 6, 2011. http://wholerawfoodnow.com/articles/item/23-diet-soda-dilemma Accessed Jan. 22, 2014.

7. America Nutrition Association. *Low Grade, Chronic Acidosis...What in the CELL is going on?* May 1,

2012. http://americannutritionassociation.org/blog/ph-life/05_01_2012/low-grade-chronic-acidosiswhat-cell-going Accessed Jan. 22, 2014.

8. Oberg, Mary. *AminoSweet -- a New Name for Aspartame.* Yahoo! Aug 24, 2010. http://voices.yahoo.com/aminosweet-name-aspartame-6653526.html?cat=70 Accessed Jan. 22, 2014.

9. Mercola DO, Joseph M. *Aspartame's Hidden Dangers.* Mercola.com. 1997-2013. http://www.mercola.com/article/aspartame/hidden_dangers.htm Accessed Jan. 22, 2014.

10. Whole Health Associates. *Aspartame: What You Should Know.* http://www.wholehealthassoc.com/aspartame.html Accessed Jan. 22, 2014.

11. Dach M.D., Jeffrey. *Diet Sodas, Aspartame, Migraine, Seizures, Brain Tumors and Stroke.* Jeffrey Dach MD Bioldentical Hormone Blog. February 13, 2011. http://jeffreydach.com/2011/02/13/diet-sodas-aspartame-stroke-jeffreydachmd.aspx Accessed Jan. 22, 2014.

12. Mission Possible World Health International. February 13, 2013. www.mpwhi.com Accessed Jan. 22, 2014.

13. Pick OB/GYN, Marcelle. *Sugar Substitutes and the Potential Danger of Splenda.* Women to Women. 1998-2013. http://www.womentowomen.com/healthyweight/splenda.aspx Accessed Jan. 22, 2014.

14. Rettner, Rachel. *How safe is Splenda? Group urges caution for artificial sweetener.* LiveScience, June 12, 2013. http://www.foxnews.com/health/2013/06/12/how-safe-is-splenda-group-urges-caution-for-artificial-sweetener/ Accessed Jan. 22, 2014.

15. Truth in Labeling Campaign. *Names of ingredients that contain processed free glutamic acid (MSG).* February 2011. http://www.truthinlabeling.org/hiddensources.html Accessed Jan. 22, 2014.

16. J.D. Heyes, Russell Blaylock MSG interview. *Dr. Russell Blaylock Reveals Secrets of MSG Toxicity (Excitotoxins) in Health Ranger interview.* March 14, 2012. NaturalNews.com, http://www.naturalnews.com/035243_

Russell_Blaylock_MSG_interview.html#ixzz2Y878BLTI Accessed Jan. 22, 2014.

17. He, Ka. Du, Shufa. Xun, Pencheng. Sharma, Sangita. Et. All. *Consumption of Monosodium Glutamate in Relation to Incidence of Overweight in Chinese adults: China Health and Nutrition Survey (CHNS)*[1,2,3]. The American Journal of Clinical Nutrition. American Society for Nutrition. The 2011. http://ajcn.nutrition.org/content/93/6/1328 Accessed Jan. 22, 2014.

18. Mission Possible World Health International. http://www.mpwhi.com/main.htm Accessed Jan. 22, 2014.

19. Med India Network for Health. *Top 12 Dangerous Additives.* http://www.medindia.net/patients/lifestyleandwellness/top-12-dangerous-food-additives.htm Accessed Jan. 22, 2014.

20. Center for Science in the Public Interest. *Chemical Cuisine, Learn about Food Additives.* http://www.cspinet.org/reports/chemcuisine.htm Accessed Jan. 22, 2014.

21. Doctoroz.com, *Food Dyes: Are They Safe?* March 13, 2013. http://www.doctoroz.com/videos/food-dyes-are-they-safe Accessed Jan. 22, 2014.

22. Hatfield, Heather. *Hidden Sources of Gluten.* WebMD.com. http://www.webmd.com/diet/features/hidden-sources-of-gluten Accessed Jan. 22, 2014.

23. Mayo Clinic. *Nutrition and Healthy Eating.* http://www.mayoclinic.com/health/gluten-free-diet/my01140 Accessed Jan. 22, 2014.

24. Ji, Sayer. *Wheat: 200 Clinically Confirmed Reasons Not to Eat It.* GreenMedInfo, Education Equals Empowerment. October 7, 2012. http://www.greenmedinfo.com/content/wheat-200-clinically-confirmed-reasons-not-eat-it Accessed Jan. 22, 2014.

25. Ford Dr., Rodney. *Gluten: Bad for Us All!* GreenMedInfo, Education Equals Empowerment. January 22, 2012. http://www.greenmedinfo.com/blog/gluten-bad-us-all Accessed Jan. 22, 2014.

26. Cochran, Amanda. *Modern Wheat a "perfect, chronic poison," Doctor Says.* CBS News. September 3, 2012.

http://www.cbsnews.com/2102-505269_162-57505149.
html Accessed Jan. 22, 2014.

27. Dr. Davis, William. *The Gliadin Effect.* Wheat Belly. January 14, 2012. http://www.wheatbellyblog. com/2012/01/the-gliadin-effect/ Accessed Jan. 22, 2014.

28. Ji, Sayer. *Wheat Contains Not One, but 23K Potentially Harmful Proteins.* GreenMedInfo, Education Equals Empowerment. October 12, 2012. http://www. greenmedinfo.com/blog/wheat-contains-not-one-23k-potentially-harmful-proteins Accessed Jan. 22, 2014.

29. Cochran, Amanda. *Modern Wheat a "perfect, chronic poison," Doctor Says.* CBS News. September 3, 2012. http://www.cbsnews.com/2102-505269_162-57505149. html Accessed Jan. 22, 2014.

30. Shewry, Peter R., Halford, Nigel G., Belton, Peter S., et. all *The Structure and Properties of Gluten: An Elastic Protein from Wheat Grain.* PMC US National Library of Medicine National Institutes of Health. February 28, 2002. http://www.ncbi.nlm.nih.gov/pmc/articles/ PMC1692935/ Accessed Jan. 22, 2014.

31. Veraverbeke, WS. Delcour, JA. *Wheat Protein Composition and Properties of Wheat Glutenin in Relation to Breadmaking Functionality.* PubMed. gov. http://www.ncbi.nlm.nih.gov/pubmed/12058979 Accessed Jan. 22, 2014.

32. Ji, Sayer. *Opening Pandora's Bread Box: The Critical Role of Wheat Lectin in Human Disease.* GreenMedInfo Education Equals Empowerment. http://www. greenmedinfo.com/page/opening-pandoras-bread-box-critical-role-wheat-lectin-human-disease Accessed Jan. 22, 2014.

33. Ford Dr., Rodney. *Gluten: Bad for Us All!* GreenMedInfo, Education Equals Empowerment. January 22, 2012. http://www.greenmedinfo.com/blog/gluten-bad-us-all Accessed Jan. 22, 2014.

34. PubMed Health. *Celiac Disease – Sprue.* January 20, 2010. http://www.ncbi.nlm.nih.gov/pubmedhealth/

PMH0001280/ Accessed Jan. 22, 2014.

35. Nordqvist, Christian. *What is Gluten Intolerance? What is Celiac Disease?* Medical News Today. April 26, 2012. http://www.medicalnewstoday.com/articles/38085.php Accessed Jan. 22, 2014.

36. Gluten Free Works. *Gluten Sensitivity.* 2011. http://glutenfreeworks.com/gluten-disorders/gluten-sensitivity/ Accessed Jan. 22, 2014.

37. Beck, Melinda. *Clues to Gluten Sensitivity.* The Wall Street Journal. March 15, 2011. http://online.wsj.com/article/SB10001424052748704893604576200393522456636.html# Accessed Jan. 22, 2014.

38. U.S. Department of Health and Human Services. *Lactose Intolerance.* National Digestive Diseases Information Clearinghouse (NDDIC). April 23, 2012. http://digestive.niddk.nih.gov/ddiseases/pubs/lactoseintolerance/ Accessed Jan. 22, 2014. **38a.** O'Neil, Dennis. *Lactose Intolerance.* Human Biological Adaptability: An Introduction to Human Responses to Common Environmental Stresses. http://anthro.palomar.edu/adapt/adapt_5.htm Accessed Jan. 22, 2014.

39. Body Ecology. *Are You Sensitive to Casein in Dairy and Don't Even Know It?* November 9, 2006. http://bodyecology.com/articles/sensitive_to_casein_in_dairy.php Accessed Jan. 22, 2014.

40. Winslow, Amelia. *Lactose Intolerant? What Can You Eat?* Eating Made Easy. March 26, 2011. http://eating-made-easy.com/2011/03/26/lactose-intolerant-what-can-you-eat/ Accessed Jan. 22, 2014.

41. Ellen's Kitchen. *Non-Dairy Sources of Calcium.* 1998-2012. http://www.ellenskitchen.com/faqs/calcium.html Accessed Jan. 22, 2014.

42. Be Food Smart. *Monoglycerides.* August 19, 2010. http://www.befoodsmart.com/ingredients/monoglycerides.php Accessed Jan. 22, 2014.

43. Dhibi M, Brahmi F, Mnari A, et. all. *The intake of high fat diet with different trans fatty acid levels differentially induces oxidative stress and non alcoholic fatty liver*

disease (NAFLD) in rats. PubMed.com. September 2013. http://www.ncbi.nlm.nih.gov/pubmed/21943357 Accessed Jan. 22, 2014.

44. Stossel, Richard. *Why Hydrogenated Oils Should Be Avoided at All Costs.* Natural News.com. November 04, 2008. http://www.naturalnews.com/024694_oil_food_oils.html Accessed Jan. 22, 2014.

45. Adams, Mike. *How Partially-Hydrogenated Oils and Trans Fats Destroy your Health.* Natural News. com. November 10, 2009. http://www.naturalnews.com/027445_fat_fats_trans.html Accessed Jan. 22, 2014.

46. Adams, Mike. *Dangers of Hydrogenated Oils Revealed in New Downloadable Report (press release).* Natural News.com. July 27, 2005. http://www.naturalnews.com/010095_hydrogenated_oils_unhealthy.html Accessed Jan. 22, 2014.

47. Dean, Deanna. *Nightshade Vegetables may Cause Adverse Reactions in Some People.* Natural News. com. January 20, 2010. http://www.naturalnews.com/027978_nightshade_vegetables.html Accessed Jan. 22, 2014.

48. Childers Ph.D., Norman. *The Nightshades.* Arthritis Nightshades Research Foundation. http://www.noarthritis.com/nightshades.htm Accessed Jan. 22, 2014.

49. Pick OB/GYN, Marcelle. *Thyroid Health.* Women to Women. May 27, 2011. http://www.womentowomen.com/hypothyroidism/goitrogenicfoods-thyroidhealth.aspx Accessed Jan. 22, 2014.

50. Pick OB/GYN, Marcelle. *Thyroid Health.* Women to Women. May 27, 2011. http://www.womentowomen.com/hypothyroidism/goitrogenicfoods-thyroidhealth.aspx Accessed Jan. 22, 2014.

51. The World's Healthiest Foods. *What are Goitrogens and in Which Foods are They Found?* 2001-2013. http://www.whfoods.com/genpage.php?tname=george&dbid=47 Accessed Jan. 22, 2014.

52. Division of Medical Devices. _Latex-Fruit Syndrome and Class 2 Food Allergy._ http://dmd.nihs.go.jp/latex/cross-e.html Accessed Jan. 22, 2014.

53. _Latex Allergy - Information for Health Professionals._ New York State Department of Health. May 2012. http://www.health.ny.gov/publications/1453/ Accessed Jan. 27, 2014.

54. Grier, Tom. _Cross Reactive Food._ American Latex Allergy Association. 1996-2013. http://www.latexallergyresources.org/cross-reactive-food Accessed Jan. 22, 2014.

55. New York State Department of Health. _Latex Allergy – Information for Health Professionals._ http://www.health.ny.gov/publications/1453/ Accessed Jan. 22, 2014.

56. Mayo Clinic staff. _Latex Allergy._ Mayo Clinic. November 16, 2011. http://www.mayoclinic.com/health/latex-allergy/DS00621/DSECTION=symptoms Accessed Jan. 22, 2014.

57. Grier, Tom. _Cross Reactive Food._ American Latex Allergy Association. http://www.latexallergyresources.org/cross-reactive-food Accessed Jan. 22, 2014.

Part 2, Step Two: Bring Back the Balance
Chapter 1 – The Omega 6 – Omega 3 Imbalance

1. Sullivan CN, Krispin. _Update on Essential Fats._ Krispin's Komments on Nutrition and Health. May 13, 2011. http://www.krispin.com/omega3.html#N6 Accessed Jan. 22, 2014.

2. Francis, Raymond. _Inflammation: A Common Denominator of Disease._ Arizona Center for Advanced Medicine. Originally printed in Well Being Journal, November/December 2008. REPRINTED WITH PERMISSION FROM BEYOND HEALTH® News. 2007-2013. http://www.arizonaadvancedmedicine.com/articles/inflammation_francis.html Accessed Jan. 22, 2014.

3. JMYarlott.com _Foods with High Omega-6._ Food and

Health Information. http://jmyarlott.com/omega6s/ Accessed Jan. 22, 2014.

4. NCBI PubMed.gov. *Omega-3 Fatty Acids EPA and DHA: Health Benefits Throughout Life.* January, 2012. http://www.ncbi.nlm.nih.gov/pubmed/22332096 Accessed Jan. 22, 2014.

5. Green Med Info.com *A Lower Ratio of Omega-6/ Omega-3 Fatty Acids is Needed for the Prevention and Management of Chronic Diseases.* Education Equals Empowerment. 2008-2013. http://www.greenmedinfo. com/search/gmi/Omega%203 Accessed Jan. 22, 2014.

6. Dr. Sears, William. *Omega-3 and DHA as Brain Food.* AskDrSears.com http://www.askdrsears.com/topics/ family-nutrition/dha/dha-brain-food Accessed Jan. 22, 2014.

7. University of Maryland Medical Center. *Omega-3 Fatty Acids.* May 10, 2011. http://www.umm.edu/altmed/ articles/omega-3-000316.htm#ixzz2JwyvjiRB Accessed Jan. 22, 2014.

8. Norris RD, Jack. *Omega-3 Fatty Acid Recommendations for Vegetarians.* VeganHealth.org. May 2012 http://www. veganhealth.org/articles/omega3 Accessed Jan. 22, 2014.

9. Morris, Eric. *Algae is your New Friend.* Super Hero News, Adventures in Becoming Superhuman. March 29, 2011. http://eric-morris.com/?p=171 Accessed Jan. 22, 2014.

10. Mercola DO. Joseph M. *The Science is Practically Screaming... Don't Make This Trendy Fat Mistake.* Dr. Mercola. November 11, 2011, http://articles.mercola. com/sites/articles/archive/2011/11/11/everything-you-need-to-know-about-fatty-acids.aspx Accessed Jan. 22, 2014.

11. The Nutrition Source. *Harvard School of Public Health. Fats and Cholesterol: Out with the bad, in with the good.* http://www.hsph.harvard.edu/nutritionsource/fats-full-story/ Accessed Jan. 22, 2014.

12. Dr. Muneeb Younus, Syed. *What Are Healthy Fats?*

Pati Chandler

Medical News Today. July 24, 2008 http://www.medicalnewstoday.com/articles/115936.php Accessed Jan. 22, 2014.

Chapter 2 – The Calcium – Magnesium Imbalance

1. Dr. Dean, Carolyn. *The Calcium Wars: Magnesium Deficiency Causes Heart Disease.* Natural News.com. December 9, 2012. http://www.naturalnews.com/038286_magnesium_deficiency_heart_disease.html Accessed Jan. 22, 2014.
2. Sears MD, Al. *Calcium Supplements Don't Build Strong Bones.* Alsearsmd.com, November 3, 2009 http://www.alsearsmd.com/calcium-supplements-bones/ Accessed Jan. 22, 2014.
3. Campbell Ph.D., Colin T. *China Report: Osteoporosis.* T. Colin Campbell Foundation. 2008. http://www.tcolincampbell.org/courses-resources/article/china-report-osteoporosis/category/bone-joint-connective-tissue-and-rheumatic-disease-1/?tx_ttnews%5BbackPid%5D=76&cHash=f19269ebbe73ea1bdb821c-828810d37c Accessed Jan. 22, 2014.
4. Well Being Journal. 1992-2002. www.wellbeingjournal.com Accessed Jan. 22, 2014.
5. Dr. Dean, Carolyn. *The Calcium Wars: Magnesium Deficiency Causes Heart Disease.* Natural News.com. December 09, 2012. http://www.naturalnews.com/038286_magnesium_deficiency_heart_disease.html Accessed Jan. 22, 2014.
6. Fuchs Ph.D., Nan Kathryn. *Magnesium: A Key to Calcium Absorption.* The Magnesium Web Site, Magnesium Online Library. November 22, 2002. http://www.mgwater.com/calmagab.shtml Accessed Jan. 22, 2014.
7. Ikeda T, Kimura S, Imazawa T, et. all. *Effects of Dietary Magnesium Deficiency in the Rat: with Special Reference to Ultrastructural Examination.* NCBI Pub Med.gov, 1997. http://www.ncbi.nlm.nih.gov/pubmed/9641824 Accessed Jan. 22, 2014.

8. Bigi A, Compostella L, Fichera AM, et. all. *Structural and Chemical Characterization of Inorganic Deposits in Calcified Human Mitral Valve.* NCBI Pub Med. gov., October, 1988. http://www.ncbi.nlm.nih.gov/pubmed/?term=3199134 Accessed Jan. 22, 2014.

9. Steidl L, Ditmar R. *Soft Tissue Calcification Treated with Local and Oral Magnesium Therapy.* June 3, 1990. NCBI Pub Med.gov. http://www.ncbi.nlm.nih.gov/pubmed/?term=2133625 Accessed Jan. 22, 2014.

10. Sircus Ac., OMD, Mark. *The Importance of Staving Off a Magnesium Deficiency.* May 09, 2008. Natural News. com. http://www.naturalnews.com/023199_magnesium_food_medicine.html Accessed Jan. 22, 2014.

11. *Magnesium.* University of Maryland Medical Center. http://umm.edu/health/medical/altmed/supplement/magnesium Accessed Jan. 22, 2014.

12. *Magnesium.* University of Maryland Medical Center. http://umm.edu/health/medical/altmed/supplement/magnesium Accessed Jan. 22, 2014.

13. *Magnesium.* University of Maryland Medical Center. http://umm.edu/health/medical/altmed/supplement/magnesium Accessed Jan. 22, 2014.

14. Dr. Mark Sircus, Ac., OMD, DM, *Magnesium Deficiency Symptoms and Diagnosis* DrSircus.com, http://drsircus.com/medicine/magnesium/magnesium-deficiency-symptoms-diagnosis Accessed Jan. 27, 2014.

15. Macri, Irena. *Paleo & Calcium, Friendly Calcium Rich Foods.* Eat & Drink Paleo. http://eatdrinkpaleo.com.au/paleo-diet-calcium-non-dairy-calcium-rich-foods/ Accessed Jan. 29. 2014.

16. Office of Dietary Supplements National Institutes of Health. *Dietary Supplement Fact Sheet: Magnesium.* http://ods.od.nih.gov/factsheets/Magnesium-HealthProfessional/ Accessed Jan. 22, 2014.

Chapter 3 – The Acid – Alkaline Imbalance

1. http://www.dummies.com/how-to/content/how-

homeostasis-keeps-your-system-in-balance.html
Accessed Jan. 22, 2014.

2. Domenico Dr., Phil. *The Acid-Alkaline Food Guide: Interview with the Author.* July 24, 2008. Natural News. com. http://www.naturalnews.com/023694_food_foods_ health.html Accessed Jan. 22, 2014.

3. *Acid Alkaline Imbalance.* pH Balance. http://www. naturalhealthschool.com/pH-balance.html Accessed Jan. 22, 2014.

4. Cancer Fighting Strategies. *pH and Cancer: Acidic pH Levels Can Lead to Cancer...Normalizing pH Levels Can Stop Cancer in its Tracks.* http://www. cancerfightingstrategies.com/ph-and-cancer.html Accessed Jan. 22, 2014.

5. Crohns.net. *Alkaline and Acid Food Charts.* http://www. crohns.net/Miva/education/acid_alkaline_foods.shtml Accessed Jan. 22, 2014.

6. Alkaline-alkaline.com. *Food pH Chart – Most Alkaline and Acidic Foods.* http://www.alkaline-alkaline.com/ph_ food_chart.html Accessed Jan. 22, 2014.

7. http://www.betterhealththruresearch.com/SodaPop.htm Accessed Jan. 22, 2014.

8. Natural-Cancer-Treatment.com *List of Alkaline-Acid Ash-Forming Foods.* http://www.natural-cancer-treatment. com/Alkaline-Acid.html Accessed Jan. 22, 2014.

9. *A list of Acid/Alkaline Forming Foods.* http://rense. com/1.mpicons/acidalka.htm Accessed Jan. 22, 2014.

10. PRWEB. *Introducing Alkaline Water Drops – pH Booster Drops Balance the pH in Water.* December 14, 2011. http://www.prweb.com/releases/alkaline-water-drops/ ph-booster-pods/prweb9020563.htm Accessed Jan. 22, 2014.

11. Fit4Maui.com. *pH of Popular Bottled Water.* http:// fit4maui.com/water/pu/bottled_ph.html Accessed Jan. 22, 2014.

Part 3, Step Three: Start Putting Out the Fire with Healthy Nutritious Food

Chapter 1 – The Relationship between Food and Pain

1. U.S. News. *Best Diets Overall.* Health, Health & Wellness. http://health.usnews.com/best-diet/best-overall-diets Accessed Jan. 27, 2014.
2. Mayo Clinic Staff. *Mediterranean diet: A Heart-Healthy Eating Plan.* Mayo Clinic. http://www.mayoclinic.com/health/mediterranean-diet/CL00011 Accessed Jan. 22, 2014.
3. Caveman Power. *The Caveman Power Diet.* http://www.cavemanpower.com/food/caveman_power_diet.html Accessed Jan. 27, 2014.
4. Lear, Jane. *Jane Says: The 'Food Combining' Diet –Fact, Fiction, or Something in Between?* Take Part. September 26, 2012. http://www.takepart.com/article/2012/09/26/jane-says-lets-look-science-behind-food-combining-trend Accessed Jan. 27, 2014.
5. Food Combing Diet. *Welcome to the "Food Combining Diet."* www.food-combining-diet.com Accessed Jan. 27, 2014.
6. Lear, Jane. *Jane Says: The 'Food Combining' Diet –Fact, fiction, or Something in Between?* Take Part. September 26, 2012. http://www.takepart.com/article/2012/09/26/jane-says-lets-look-science-behind-food-combining-trend Accessed Jan. 27, 2014.

Chapter 2 – Those Important "Little Things."

1. Hadhazy, Adam. *Think Twice: How the Gut's 'Second Brain' Influences Mood and Well-Being.* Scientific American. February 24, 2010. http://www.scientificamerican.com/article.cfm?id=gut-second-brain Accessed Jan. 27, 2014.
2. Campbell-McBride, MD., *GAPSTM*, Natasha. DoctorNatasha.com. http://www.doctor-natasha.com/gaps-book.php Accessed Jan. 27, 2014.
3. Mercola, Joseph M. *The Type of Food That Will Slow Nearly Every Inflammatory Disease.* Mercola.com.

August 21, 2001. http://articles.mercola.com/sites/
articles/archive/2011/08/21/enzymes-special-report.aspx
Accessed Jan. 27, 2014.

4. Mercola DO, Joseph M. *The Type of Food That Will
Slow Nearly Every Inflammatory Disease.* Mercola.
com. August 21, 2001. http://articles.mercola.com/sites/
articles/archive/2011/08/21/enzymes-special-report.aspx
Accessed Jan. 27, 2014.

5. Harder, Ron. *The Power of Enzymes.* Thyroid
Newsroom. Thyroid Disease. About.com. October 2001.
http://thyroid.about.com/library/news/blenzymes.htm
Accessed Jan. 27, 2014.

6. Ron. *The Power of Enzymes.* Thyroid Newsroom.
Thyroid Disease. About.com. October 2001. http://
thyroid.about.com/library/news/blenzymes.htm
Accessed Jan. 27, 2014.

7. Gluten Free Works. *Gluten Sensitivity.* http://
glutenfreeworks.com/gluten-disorders/gluten-sensitivity/
Accessed Jan. 27, 2014.

8. Ji, Sayer. *Wheat Contains Not One, but 23K Potentially
Harmful Proteins.* GreenMedInfo. October 12, 2012.
http://www.greenmedinfo.com/blog/wheat-contains-not-
one-23k-potentially-harmful-proteins Accessed Jan. 27,
2014.

9. Barron, Jon. *Proteolytic Enzymes.* Nutritional Wellness.
http://www.nutritionalwellness.com/archives/2006/jul/07_
proteolytic.php Accessed Jan. 27, 2014.

10. Gonzales MD., Nicholas. *Enzyme Therapy and Cancer.*
Dr-Gonzales.com. http://www.dr-gonzalez.com/history_
of_treatment.htm Accessed Jan. 27, 2014.

11. Global Healing Center. *The Health Benefits of Amylase.*
October 11, 2013. http://www.globalhealingcenter.com/
natural-health/the-health-benefits-of-amylase/ Accessed
Jan. 27, 2014.

12. World of Enzymes and Probiotics. *Lipase.* http://
worldofenzymes.info/enzymes-introduction/lipase/
Accessed Jan. 27, 2014.

13. Monarch, Matt. *Extend Your Life with Enzymes.*

NaturalNews.com. January 17, 2009. http://www.
naturalnews.com/022511_junk_food_All_Jacked_
Up.html Accessed Jan. 27, 2014.

14. Barron, Jon. *Proteolytic Enzymes.* Nutritional Wellness.
    http://www.nutritionalwellness.com/archives/2006/jul/07_
    proteolytic.php Accessed Jan. 27, 2014.

15. Wisegeek. *What are Metabolic Enzymes?* http://www.
    wisegeek.com/what-are-metabolic-enzymes.htm
    Accessed Jan. 27, 2014.

16. Lous, PF. *Digestive Enzymes Enhance Nutrient
    Absorption, Gut Health and Longevity.* NaturalNews.
    com. August 7, 2012. http://www.naturalnews.
    com/036717_digestive_enzymes_nutrient_absorption_
    longevity.html Accessed Jan. 27, 2014.

17. Fallon, Sally. Enig PhD, Mary G., The Weston A. Price
    Foundation® for Wise Traditions in Food, Farming and
    Healing Arts. January 1, 2000, http://www.westonaprice.
    org/nutrition-greats/edward-howell Accessed Jan. 27,
    2014.

18. Dr. Jockers, David. *Boosting Your Enzyme Reserves.*
    NaturalNews.com, October 20, 2012. http://www.
    naturalnews.com/037607_enzymes_digestion_nutrient_
    assimilation.html Accessed Jan. 27, 2014.

19. NYU Langone Medical Center. *Proteolytic Enzymes.*
    http://www.med.nyu.edu/content?ChunkIID=21671_
    Accessed Jan. 27, 2014.

20. Dr. Jockers, David. *Start Your Day with Water and
    Lemon.* NaturalNews.com. November 27, 2011. http://
    www.naturalnews.com/034249_lemon_juice_energy.
    html Accessed Jan. 27, 2014.

21. Heustad, R.N., Ann *The Amazing Health Benefits
    of Drinking Lemon Water.* Proliberty.com. The
    Idaho Observer. July 2004. http://proliberty.com/
    observer/20040711.htm Accessed Jan. 27, 2014.

22. Global Healing Center. *The Health Benefits of Probiotics.*
    May 11, 2009. http://www.globalhealingcenter.com/
    natural-health/health-benefits-of-probiotics/ Accessed
    Jan. 27, 2014.

23. Mercola DO, Joseph M. *Probiotics Found to Your Gut's Immune System.* Mercola.com. 5, 2008. http://articles.mercola.com/sites/articles/archive/2008/07/05/probiotics-found-to-help-your-gut-s-immune-system.aspx Accessed Jan. 27, 2014.

24. Adams, Case. *Probiotics Change Brain Activity, Emotional Response.* GreenMedInfo. March 22, 2013. http://www.greenmedinfo.com/blog/probiotics-change-brain-activity-emotional-response?utm_source=www.GreenMedInfo.com&utm_campaign=d107459109-Greenmedinfo&utm_medium=email Accessed Jan. 27, 2014.

25. Probiotics.org. http://probiotics.org/amazing-facts/ Accessed Jan. 27, 2014.

26. Adams, Casey. *The Promising Potential of Prebiotics & Probiotics.* Nutraceuticals World. May 1, 2009. http://www.nutraceuticalsworld.com/issues/2009-05/view_features/the-promising-potential-of-prebiotics-amp-probioti/ Accessed Jan. 27, 2014.

27. Seeley, Merlyn. *America's 10 Best Foods: Unsweetened Yogurt.* Natural Living Examiner. Examiner.com. February 14, 2011. http://www.examiner.com/article/america-s-10-best-foods-unsweetened-yogurt Accessed Jan. 27, 2014.

28. Seeley, Merlyn. *America's 10 Best Foods: Unsweetened Yogurt.* Natural Living Examiner. Examiner.com. February 14, 2011. http://www.examiner.com/article/america-s-10-best-foods-unsweetened-yogurt Accessed Jan. 27, 2014.

29. Anjali. *Grocery Store Guide: Navigating the Yogurt Aisle.* The Picky Eater. April 15, 2013. http://pickyeaterblog.com/grocery-store-guide-navigating-the-yogurt-aisle/ Accessed Jan. 27, 2014.

30. DietDoctor.com. *Why Americans are Obese: Nonfat Yogurt.* July 7, 2011. http://www.dietdoctor.com/why-americans-are-obese-nonfat-yogurt Accessed Jan. 27, 2014 and **30a**. Burkett, Eric. *Low-fat yogurt: why bother?* Food Examiner. Examiner.com. April 7, 2009. http://

www.examiner.com/article/low-fat-yogurt-why-bother Accessed Jan. 27, 2014.

31. Dr. Sears, William. *10 Reasons Yogurt is a Top Health Food.* AskDrSears.com. http://www.askdrsears.com/topics/family-nutrition/yogurt/10-reasons-yogurt-top-health-food Accessed Jan. 27, 2014.

32. Main, Emily. *The truth about probiotics.* Rodale News. http://www.rodalenews.com/probiotic-foods Accessed Jan. 27, 2014.

33. Probiotic Foods. *What are Probiotics?* Global Healing Center. January, 21, 2011. http://www.globalhealingcenter.com/natural-health/probiotic-foods/ Accessed Jan. 27, 2014.

34. Sisson, Mark. *The Definitive Guide to Fermented Foods.* Mark's Daily Apple. http://www.marksdailyapple.com/fermented-foods-health/#axzz2TBYMkZyS Accessed Jan. 27, 2014.

35. Adams, Casey. *The Promising Potential of Prebiotics & Probiotics.* Nutraceuticals World. May 1, 2009. http://www.nutraceuticalsworld.com/issues/2009-05/view_features/the-promising-potential-of-prebiotics-amp-probioti/ Accessed Jan. 27, 2014.

36. Probiotics.org. http://probiotics.org/amazing-facts/ Accessed Jan. 27, 2014.

37. Miller, Zach C. *Health is Directly Linked to the Gut: Eleven Things That Destroy the Beneficial Probiotic Bacteria Living Inside Us.* NaturalNews.com. May 3, 2013. http://www.naturalnews.com/040353_friendly_bacteria_foods_gut_health.html Accessed Jan. 27, 2014.

38. www.ConsumerLab.com Accessed Jan. 27, 2014.

39. Enzymestuff. *What to Look for in a Probiotic.* The probiotic short-course. http://www.enzymestuff.com/probiotics.htm Accessed Jan. 27, 2014.

40. NYU Langone Medical Center. *Acidophilus and Other Probiotics.* http://www.med.nyu.edu/content?ChunkIID=21454 Accessed Jan. 27, 2014.

41. Haupt, Angela. Hiatt, Kurtis. *Greek Yogurt vs. Regular*

Yogurt: Which is More Healthful? US News. Health. September 30, 2011. http://health.usnews.com/health-news/diet-fitness/diet/articles/2011/09/30/greek-yogurt-vs-regular-yogurt-which-is-more-healthful Accessed Jan. 27, 2014.

42. Jetvig MS, Shereen. *Probiotics and the Prebiotics that Feed Them, For a Happy Gut.* About.com. December 25, 2013. http://nutrition.about.com/od/therapeuticnutrition1/p/pro_prebiotics.htm Accessed Jan. 27, 2014.

43. McKinney, M.S., R.D., L.D.N., C.D.E., Christine. *The Benefits of Prebiotics.* Yahoo Health. July 28, 2012. http://health.yahoo.net/experts/livingwithdiabetes/benefits-prebiotics Accessed Jan. 27, 2014.

44. Best Prebiotic Supplement. *What are Prebiotics.* http://best-prebiotic-supplement.com/ Accessed Jan. 27, 2014.

45. Brownawell, AM. Caers, W. Gibson, GR. Kendall, et. all. *Prebiotics and the Health Benefits of Fiber: Current Regulatory Status, Future Research, and Goals.* JL. PubMed.gov. May 2012. Epub March 28, 2012. http://www.ncbi.nlm.nih.gov/pubmed/22457389 Accessed Jan. 27, 2014.

Chapter 3 – Proteins

1. DietaryFiberFoods.com. *Protein: Health Benefits, Deficiency, Sources of Protein.* http://www.dietaryfiberfood.com/protein/protein-health-benefits.php Accessed Jan. 27, 2014.

2. Bruso. Jessica *What Nutrients Consist of Essential Amino Acids & Nonessential Amino Acids?* Demand Media. SFGate. http://healthyeating.sfgate.com/nutrients-consist-essential-amino-acids-nonessential-amino-acids-3627.html Accessed Jan. 27, 2014.

3. DietaryFiberFoods.com. *Non-Essential Amino Acids: Definition and Functions.* http://www.dietaryfiberfood.com/amino-acids/non-essential-amino-acids.php

Accessed Jan. 27, 2014.

4. Stoll MD, Scott. *Yes, Plants Have Protein.* Whole Story. January 15, 2013. http://www.wholefoodsmarket.com/blog/whole-story/yes-plants-have-protein Accessed Jan. 27, 2014.

5. Benson, Jonathan. *Wheat Contains Over 23,000 Potentially Harmful Proteins.* NaturalNews.com. May 29, 2013. http://www.naturalnews.com/040538_wheat_gluten_proteins.html Accessed Jan. 27, 2014.

6. The World's Healthiest Foods. *What's New and Beneficial about Quinoa.* Quinoa. http://www.whfoods.com/genpage.php?dbid=142&tname=foodspice Accessed Jan. 27, 2014.

7. The Ohio State University. Ohio Agricultural Research and Development Center. *Chow Line: 'Mother Grain' Quinoa a Complete Protein.* Welcome to OARDC. September 26, 2008. http://oardc.osu.edu/6060/Chow-Line-Mother-grain-quinoa-a-complete-protein-(for-10/5/08).htm Accessed Jan. 27, 2014.

8. Whole Grains Council. *What is a Whole Grain?* http://wholegrainscouncil.org/whole-grains-101/what-is-a-whole-grain Accessed Jan. 27, 2014.

9. Foster, Karen. *12 Reasons to Eat Sprouts, a Living Food with Amazing Health Benefits.* PreventDisease.com. March 4, 2013. http://preventdisease.com/news/13/030413_12-Reasons-To-Eat-Sprouts-Living-Food-With-Amazing-Health-Benefits.shtml Accessed Jan. 27, 2014.

10. Whole Grains Council. *Sprouted Whole Grains.* http://wholegrainscouncil.org/whole-grains-101/sprouted-whole-grains Accessed Jan. 27, 2014.

11. Foster, Karen. *12 Reasons to Eat Sprouts, a Living Food with Amazing Health Benefits.* PreventDisease.com. March 4, 2013. http://preventdisease.com/news/13/030413_12-Reasons-To-Eat-Sprouts-Living-Food-With-Amazing-Health-Benefits.shtml Accessed Jan. 27, 2014.

12. Food for Life Baking Company. *The Sprouted Grain*

Difference™. Sprouted for Life!™. http://www.foodforlife.com/about_us/sprouted-grain-difference Accessed Jan. 27, 2014.

13. Mercola DO, Joseph. *Got Thyroid Problems? Then Stop Consuming this "Healthy" Food.* Mercola.com http://articles.mercola.com/sites/articles/archive/2010/10/13/soy-controversy-and-health-effects.aspx Accessed Jan. 27, 2014.

14. Godman, Heidi. *Extra Protein is a Decent Dietary Choice, but Don't Overdo It.* Harvard Health Letter. Harvard Health Publications. Harvard Medical School. May 1, 2013. http://www.health.harvard.edu/blog/extra-protein-is-a-decent-dietary-choice-but-dont-overdo-it-201305016145 Accessed Jan. 27, 2014.

15. Centers for Disease Control and Prevention. *Protein.* Nutrition for Everyone. http://www.cdc.gov/nutrition/everyone/basics/protein.html Accessed Jan. 27, 2014.

16. Conrad-Stoppler MD, Melissa. Balentine DO, Jerry R. *How Much Dietary Protein Should People Consume?* MedicineNet.com. http://www.medicinenet.com/script/main/art.asp?articlekey=50900 Accessed Jan. 27, 2014.

17. MedlinePlus. *Protein in Diet.* http://www.nlm.nih.gov/medlineplus/ency/article/002467.htm Accessed Jan. 27, 2014.

18. MedlinePlus. *Protein in Diet.* http://www.nlm.nih.gov/medlineplus/ency/article/002467.htm Accessed Jan. 27, 2014.

19. The World's healthiest foods. *A New Way of Looking at Proteins, Fats and Carbohydrates.* http://www.whfoods.com/genpage.php?tname=faq&dbid=7 Accessed Jan. 27, 2014.

20. Conrad-Stoppler MD, Melissa. Balentine DO, Jerry R. *How Much Dietary Protein Should People Consume?* MedicineNet.com. http://www.medicinenet.com/script/main/art.asp?articlekey=50900 Accessed Jan. 27, 2014.

21. Conrad-Stoppler MD, Melissa. Balentine DO, Jerry R. *How Much Dietary Protein Should People Consume?* MedicineNet.com. http://www.medicinenet.com/script/

main/art.asp?articlekey=50900 Accessed Jan. 27, 2014.

22. Jaffe MD, PhD, Russell M. *An MD's Perspective on How to Avoid, Treat and Reverse Diabetes.* GreenMedInfo. May 31, 2013. http://www.greenmedinfo.com/blog/mds-perspective-how-avoid-treat-and-reverse-diabetes Accessed Jan. 27, 2014.

23. Conrad-Stoppler MD, Melissa. Balentine DO, Jerry R. *How Much Dietary Protein Should People Consume?* MedicineNet.com. http://www.medicinenet.com/script/main/art.asp?articlekey=50900 Accessed Jan. 27, 2014.

24. Collins MD, Richard. *Balance Carbs, Protein and Fat for Better Health.* The Cooking Cardiologist. June 23, 2011. http://www.thecookingcardiologist.com/cardiologist-blog/balance-carbs-protein-and-fat-better-health Accessed Jan. 27, 2014.

Chapter 4 – Fats

1. Huffpost Healthy Living. *Why Do We Overeat? Harvard Researchers Address Obesity and the Toxic Food Environment.* Huffington Post. September 13, 2013. http://www.huffingtonpost.com/2013/09/13/why-we-overeat_n_3919317.html?utm_hp_ref=mostpopular Accessed Jan. 27, 2014.

2. Jaslow, Ryan. *5 Percent of U.S. Kids "Severely Obese," Warns American Heart Association.* CBS News. September 10, 2013. http://www.cbsnews.com/8301-204_162-57602071/5-percent-of-u.s-kids-severely-obese-warns-american-heart-association/ Accessed Jan. 27, 2014.

3. Mercola DO, Joseph M. *The Hypocrisy of Federal Fitness Promotions.* Mercola.com. September 27, 2013. http://fitness.mercola.com/sites/fitness/archive/2013/09/27/federal-fitness-promotions.aspx?e_cid=20130927Z1_DNL_art_1&utm_source=dnl&utm_medium=email&utm_content=art1&utm_campaign=20130927Z1 Accessed Jan. 27, 2014.

4. Huff, Ethan A. *Sweden Rejects Low-Fat Diet Myth,*

Encourages Citizens to Cut Carbs and Eat More Fat. NaturalNews.com. November 5, 2013. http://www. naturalnews.com/042780_sweden_low-fat_diet_myth_ butter.html#ixzz2k4GyUoOa Accessed Jan. 27, 2014.

5. The Nutrition Source. *Fats and Cholesterol: Out With the Bad, in with the Good.* Harvard School of Public Health. http://www.hsph.harvard.edu/nutritionsource/fats-full-story/ Accessed Jan. 27, 2014.

6. The Nutrition Source. *Fats and Cholesterol: Out With the Bad, in with the Good.* Harvard School of Public Health. http://www.hsph.harvard.edu/nutritionsource/fats-full-story/ Accessed Jan. 27, 2014.

7. Challem, Jack. *A Big Fat Mistake.* Experience Life. June 2011. http://experiencelife.com/article/a-big-fat-mistake/ Accessed Jan. 27, 2014.

8. Challem, Jack. *A Big Fat Mistake.* Experience Life. June 2011. http://experiencelife.com/article/a-big-fat-mistake/ Accessed Jan. 27, 2014.

9. Dr. Muneeb-Younus, Syed. *What are Healthy Fats?* MNT. July 24, 2008. http://www.medicalnewstoday.com/articles/115936.php Accessed Jan. 27, 2014.

10. Mayo Clinic. *Dietary Fats: Know Which Types to Choose.* February 15, 2011. http://www.mayoclinic.com/health/fat/NU00262/NSECTIONGROUP=2 Accessed Jan. 27, 2014.

11. Berkey, Catherine S. Willett, Walter C. Tamimi, Rulla M. Rosner, et. all. *Vegetable Protein and Vegetable Fat Intakes in Pre-Adolescent and Adolescent Girls, and Risk for Benign Breast Disease in Young Women.* Cancer Research and Treatment. Springer Link. September 2013. http://link.springer.com/article/10.1007/s10549-013-2686-8?no-access=true Accessed Jan. 27, 2014.

12. Mercola DO, Joseph M. *Heart Specialist Calls for Major Repositioning on Saturated Fat, as it's NOT the Cause of Heart Disease.* Mercola.com. November 4, 2013. http://articles.mercola.com/sites/articles/archive/2013/11/04/saturated-fat-intake.aspx?e_cid=20131104Z1_DNL_

art_1&utm_source=dnl&utm_medium=email&utm_content=art1&utm_campaign=20131104Z1 Accessed Jan. 27, 2014.

13. Dr. Muneeb-Younus, Syed. *What are Healthy Fats?* MNT. July 24, 2008. http://www.medicalnewstoday.com/articles/115936.php Accessed Jan. 27, 2014.

14. Arizona Center for Advanced Medicine. *Chronic inflammation.* June 25, 2013. http://arizonaadvancedmedicine.com/chronic-inflammation/ Accessed Jan. 27, 2014.

15. Arizona Center for Advanced Medicine. *Chronic inflammation.* June 25, 2013. http://arizonaadvancedmedicine.com/chronic-inflammation/ Accessed Jan. 27, 2014.

16. Challem, Jack. *A Big Fat Mistake.* Experience Life. June 2011. http://experiencelife.com/article/a-big-fat-mistake/ Accessed Jan. 27, 2014.

17. Nutrition Wellness and General Nutrition. *Not All Fats are the Same.* Penn Medicine. http://www.pennmedicine.org/health_info/nutrition/not_same.html Accessed Jan. 27, 2014.

18. Donkers, Mike. *Fatal and vital foods – popular exposed.* NaturalNews.com. February 7, 2008. http://www.naturalnews.com/022608_fat_sugar_fats.html Accessed Jan. 27, 2014.

19. Medscape. http://www.medscape.com/viewarticle/574506_4 Accessed Jan. 27, 2014. and **19a.** Kontush, Anatol. Chapman, John M. *Functionally Defective High-Density Lipoprotein: A New Therapeutic Tart at the Crossroads of Dyslipidema, Inflammation, and Atherosclerosis.* Pharmacological Reviews. http://intl.pharmrev.org/content/58/3/342.full Accessed Jan. 27, 2014.

20. Merola DO, Joseph M. *Cholesterol has Benefits, Too.* Merola.com. February 2, 2008. http://articles.mercola.com/sites/articles/archive/2008/02/02/cholesterol-has-benefits-too.aspx Accessed Jan. 27, 2014.

21. Science News. *Surprise – Cholesterol May Actually*

Pose Benefits, Study Shows. ScienceDaily®.
January 10, 2008. http://www.sciencedaily.com/
releases/2008/01/080109173717.htm Accessed Jan.
27, 2014.

22. Ravnskov MD, PhD, Uffe. *The Benefits of High
Cholesterol.* The Weston A. Price Foundation. June
24, 2004. http://www.westonaprice.org/cardiovascular-
disease/benefits-of-high-cholesterol Accessed Jan. 27,
2014.

23. Ravnskov MD, PhD, Uffe. *The Benefits of High
Cholesterol.* The Weston A. Price Foundation. June
24, 2004. http://www.westonaprice.org/cardiovascular-
disease/benefits-of-high-cholesterol Accessed Jan. 27,
2014.

24. Fife N.D., Bruce. *Coconut Oil and Heart
Disease.* Coconut Research Center. http://www.
coconutresearchcenter.org/article10132.htm Accessed
Jan. 27, 2014.

25. Mattocks, Charles. *The Benefits of Coconut Oil.* The
Dr.Oz Show. October 12, 2011. http://www.doctoroz.
com/blog/charles-mattocks/benefits-coconut-oil
Accessed Jan. 27, 2014.

26. Mercola DO, Joseph M. *Which Oil Will Help you Absorb
Nutrients Better?* Mercola.com. August 20, 2012. http://
articles.mercola.com/sites/articles/archive/2012/08/20/
coconut-oil-and-saturated-fats.aspx Accessed Jan. 27,
2014.

27. Healing Naturally by Bee. *Coconut Oil for Digestive
Disorders.* http://www.healingnaturallybybee.com/
articles/coconut9.php Accessed Jan. 27, 2014.

28. Mercola DO, Joseph M. *Which Oil Will Help you Absorb
Nutrients Better?* Mercola.com. August 20, 2012. http://
articles.mercola.com/sites/articles/archive/2012/08/20/
coconut-oil-and-saturated-fats.aspx Accessed Jan. 27,
2014.

29. Ji, Sayer. *MCT Fats Found in Coconut Oil Boost Brain
Function in Only One Dose.* GreenMedInfo. http://www.
greenmedinfo.com/blog/mct-fats-found-coconut-oil-

boost-brain-function-only-one-dose?utm_source=www. GreenMedInfo.com&utm_campaign=9f5b6ae832-Greenmedinfo&utm_medium=email&utm_term=0_193c8492fb-9f5b6ae832-86761662 Accessed Jan. 27, 2014.

30. Wright, Carolanne. NaturalNews.com. *Oil Pulling: a Cheap, Easy Effective Solution to Health Woes? Modern Research Says Yes.* May 12, 2013. http://www. naturalnews.com/040293_oil_pulling_cognitive_decline_home_remedies.html Accessed Jan. 27, 2014.

31. Tru Health. *Oil Pulling.* http://truhealth.com/2013/03/28/oil-pulling-2/ Accessed Jan. 27, 2014.

32. Oil Pulling. A Wonderful Therapy. www.OilPulling.com Accessed Jan. 27, 2014.

33. Tru Health. *Oil Pulling.* http://truhealth.com/2013/03/28/oil-pulling-2/ Accessed Jan. 27, 2014.

34. MNT. *What are the Health Benefits of Olive Oil?* September 18, 2013. http://www.medicalnewstoday.com/articles/266258.php Accessed Jan. 27, 2014.

35. The World's Healthiest Foods. *What's New and Beneficial about Extra Virgin Olive Oil?* Olive Oil, extra virgin. http://www.whfoods.com/genpage.php?tname=foodspice&dbid=132 Accessed Jan. 27, 2014.

36. Whatscookingamerica.com. *Types of Cooking Fats and Oils – Smoking Points of Fats and Oils.* http://whatscookingamerica.net/Information/CookingOilTypes.htm Accessed Jan. 27, 2014.

37. Whatscookingamerica.com. *Types of Cooking Fats and Oils – Smoking Points of Fats and Oils.* http://whatscookingamerica.net/Information/CookingOilTypes.htm Accessed Jan. 27, 2014.

38. Hensrud MD, Donald. *If Olive Oil is High in Fat, Why is it Considered Healthy?* Mayo Clinic. http://www.mayoclinic.com/health/food-and-nutrition/An01037 Accessed Jan. 27, 2014.

39. Kopf, Jamie. *Is it True that Some "Extra Virgin" Olive Oil is Fake?* ConsumerReports.org. June 19, 2013.

http://www.consumerreports.org/cro/news/2013/06/is-it-true-that-some-extra-virgin-olive-oil-is-fake/index.htm Accessed Jan. 27, 2014.

40. Aubrey, Allison. *To Get the Benefits of Olive Oil, Fresh May Be Best.* The Salt. NPR. September 30, 2013. http://www.npr.org/blogs/thesalt/2013/09/30/226844915/to-get-the-benefits-of-olive-oil-fresh-may-be-best Accessed Jan. 27, 2014.

41. Aubrey, Allison. *To Get the Benefits of Olive Oil, Gresh May Be Best.* The Salt. NPR. September 30, 2013. http://www.npr.org/blogs/thesalt/2013/09/30/226844915/to-get-the-benefits-of-olive-oil-fresh-may-be-best Accessed Jan. 27, 2014.

42. Sisson, Mark. *Is Your Olive Oil Really Olive Oil?* Mark's Daily Apple. http://www.marksdailyapple.com/is-your-olive-oil-really-olive-oil/#axzz2h8UvNNmQ Accessed Jan. 27, 2014.

43. Mercola DO, Joseph M. *The Many Health Benefits of Avocado.* Mercola.com. January 17, 2013. http://articles.mercola.com/sites/articles/archive/2013/01/17/avocado-benefits.aspx Accessed Jan. 27, 2014.

44. Avocados. *What's New and Beneficial about Avocados?* The World's Healthiest Foods. http://www.whfoods.com/genpage.php?tname=foodspice&dbid=5 Accessed Jan. 27, 2014.

45. Collier-Cool, Lisa. *Avocados: The world's Most Perfect Food?* Yahoo Health. August 13, 2013. http://health.yahoo.net/experts/dayinhealth/avocados-worlds-most-perfect-food Accessed Jan. 27, 2014.

46. Phillip, John. *Avocado Help Mediate the Inflammatory Effect of Grilled Meats to Lower Risk of Heart Disease.* NaturalNews.com. August 21, 2013. http://www.naturalnews.com/041715_avocados_grilled_meats_heart_disease.html Accessed Jan. 27, 2014.

47. Hezy. *15 Health Benefits of Avocados.* Health Onlinezine. April 20, 2011. http://www.healthonlinezine.info/health-benefits-of-avocados.html Accessed Jan. 27, 2014.

48. Avocados. *What's New and Beneficial about Avocados?* The World's Healthiest Foods. http://www.whfoods.com/genpage.php?tname=foodspice&dbid=5 Accessed Jan. 27, 2014.
49. Avocados. *What's New and Beneficial about Avocados?* The World's Healthiest Foods. http://www.whfoods.com/genpage.php?tname=foodspice&dbid=5 Accessed Jan. 27, 2014.
50. Food Network. *Great Avocado Recipes.* Avocado. http://www.foodnetwork.com/topics/avocado/index.html Accessed Jan. 27, 2014.

Chapter 5 – Carbohydrates

1. Medline Plus. *Carbohydrates.* http://www.nlm.nih.gov/medlineplus/ency/article/002469.htm Accessed Jan. 27, 2014.
2. Bellamy, Bryn. *How to Identify Foods with Carbs.* Demand Media. Healthy Eating. SFGate. http://healthyeating.sfgate.com/identify-foods-carbs-2370.html Accessed Jan. 27, 2014.
3. Coffman, Melodie Anne. *Are Peas & Corn Good Carbs?* Demand Media. Healthy Eating. SFGate. http://healthyeating.sfgate.com/peas-corn-good-carbs-4113.html Accessed Jan. 27, 2014.
4. Conis, Elena. *Ancient grains: The Best Thing Since Sliced Bread?* Los Angeles Times. February 19, 2011. http://articles.latimes.com/2011/feb/19/health/la-he-ancient-grains-20110220 Accessed Jan. 27, 2014.
5. Centers for Disease Control and Prevention. *Carbohydrates.* http://www.cdc.gov/nutrition/everyone/basics/carbs.html Accessed Jan. 27, 2014.
6. Diabeticacarbguide.com. http://www.diabeticcarbguide.com/complex-carbs-five-healthy-benefits Justhost.com. Accessed Jan. 27, 2014.
7. Rodriguez, Diana. *The Lowdown on Glycemic Load.* EverydayHealth.com. http://www.everydayhealth.com/diet-nutrition/101/nutrition-basics/the-glycemic-load.aspx

Accessed Jan. 27, 2014.

8. Harvard Health Publications. *Glycemic Index and Glycemic Load for 100+ Foods.* Harvard Medical School. http://www.health.harvard.edu/newsweek/Glycemic_index_and_glycemic_load_for_100_foods.htm Accessed Jan. 27, 2014.

9. Rodriguez, Diana. *The Lowdown on Glycemic Load.* EverydayHealth.com. http://www.everydayhealth.com/diet-nutrition/101/nutrition-basics/the-glycemic-load.aspx Accessed Jan. 27, 2014.

Chapter 6 – Antioxidants

1. WebMD.com, *Super Foods for Optimal Health.* Food & Recipes. http://webmd.com/diet/guide/antioxidants-your-immune-system-super-foods-optimal-health Accessed Jan. 27, 2014.

2. Harvard School of Public Health. *Vegetables and Fruits: Get Plenty Every Day.* The Nutrition Source. http://www.hsph.harvard.edu/nutritionsource/vegetables-full-story/ Accessed Jan. 27, 2014.

3. Lerche-Davis, Jeanie. *How Antioxidants Work. Antioxidants Minimized Damage to Your Cells from Free Radicals.* WebMD Feature. WebMD. http://www.webmd.com/food-recipes/features/how-antioxidants-work1 Accessed Jan. 27, 2014.

4. Hart, Anne. *Seniors and Athletes Rurn to Cherry Juice to Lesson Osteoarthritic Pain.* Senior Health Examiner. Examiner.com. July 6, 2012. http://www.examiner.com/article/seniors-and-athletes-turn-to-cherry-juice-to-lessen-osteoarthritic-pain Accessed Jan. 27, 2014.

5. Dr. Jockers, David. *Discover the Super-Food Power of Turmeric.* NaturalNews.com February, 23, 2011. http://www.naturalnews.com/031461_turmeric_superfood.html Accessed Jan. 27, 2014.

6. Minton, Barbara L. *Substance in Black Pepper Increases Nutrient Absorption up to Two Thousand Percent.* NaturalNews.com. November 17, 2008. http://www.

naturalnews.com/024829_piperine_curcumin_black_
pepper.html Accessed Jan. 27, 2014.
7. Medicine Hunter.com. *Holy Basil: Relieve Anxiety and
Stress Naturally.* http://medicinehunter.com/holy-basil
Accessed Jan. 27, 2014.
8. Goepp MD, Julius. *New Research on the Health Benefits
of Green Tea.* Life Extension Magazine. April 2008.
http://www.lef.org/magazine/mag2008/apr2008_New-
Research-On-The-Health-Benefits-Of-Green-Tea_01.htm
Accessed Jan. 27, 2014.
9. Examine.com *Theanine.* http://examine.com/
supplements/Theanine/ Accessed Jan. 27, 2014.

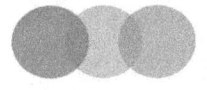

Index

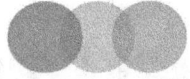

For more information or to contact the author, please visit:

Managingfibromyalgia.com
Facebook.com/pati.chandler

or

Facebook/FibromyalgiaNaturallywithPatiChandler.com

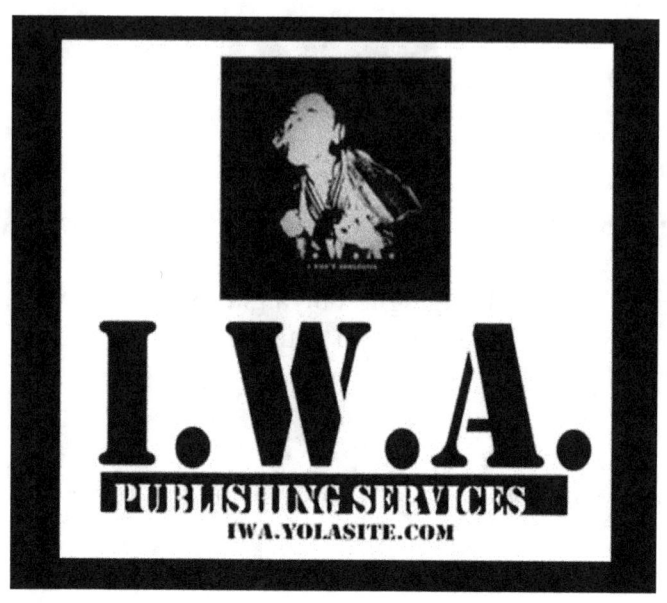

If you enjoyed reading Is *There a Diet for Chronic Illness*? Post your comments on Amazon and BN.com